Chair Massage Techniques

© 2016 Eric Brown
309- 480 Oriole Pky
Toronto, ON M5P 2H8, Canada
www.upsidebrown.net

Licensed by *Canadian Massage Training*
www.canadianmassagetraining.com

Welcome to the Certified Chair Massage Practitioner Program at *Canadian Massage Training*.

A comprehensive program to fast track you into a career as a chair massage practitioner!

Canadian Massage Training provides;

1. **In-Class training**: One-on-one in class training. Over 75 ergonomic techniques specific to the chair practitioners seated massage style. Minimal compression – maximum results to upper back, neck, shoulders, arms, and lower back is just the start of your first week.

2. **Developing Your Niche Market:** Canadian Massage Training teaches you the business side of chair massage from marketing to staffing. Connecting you with companies across Canada as well as develop your niche market, upgrade your current skill set. Begin your new career with Canadian Massage Training in 6 weeks.

3. **On-going support continues:** Connect with graduates and other practitioners through Canadian Massage Training Opportunity Board and Facebook communities. Graduates across Canada have the opportunity to join and apply for job postings from various on-site mobile companies, such as Massage on Wheels and more.

4. **Examinations, evaluations and certification:** Students must complete 15 practicum evaluations, a multiple choice exam and 2 chair massage routines; a 15 minute routine and a 10 minute routine with the instructor by the end of the program*

Students have up to 60 days after the program to complete their requirements for certification. Of the student is unable to fulfill their obligations by the end of the program. An alternative date at the convenience of the instructor and an additions fee will be applied.

Your Certification/Examination is scheduled for:

_____

*First Aid & CPR Certification classes are available to all students. Be prepared and confident as a certified chair massage practitioner and upgrade before you graduate with first aid & CPR training. Register On-line or ask your instructor for information.

A note from the author

In the early 90's I went to a workshop on marketing "on-site massage". The gentleman who developed the workshop, David Palmer, had a vision for making touch a positive social value.

Palmer had invented a portable massage chair that would allow practitioners to bring massage wherever it was convenient for the customer, whether that was their homes or their workplace. The massage would be done through the clothing to the back, neck and shoulders. This type of massage provided people a safe and accessible way to receive the benefits of positive nurturing touch.

I embraced the vision and began doing chair massage everywhere from tanning salons and bars, to tradeshows and corporate offices. I pioneered workplace massage in Canada and in particular the corporate market through my chair massage company *Relax to the Max*. Over the following years we did massage in pretty much every major tech firm, law office, hospital, and financial institution in Canada, bringing massage to thousands and thousands of people who would have never otherwise experienced the benefits of structured touch.

After 25 years of doing this valuable work, I decided to pass the torch onto other passionate practitioners. Many of these practitioners like the folks behind Canadian Massage Training continue the training tradition started by Relax to the Max to and enthusiastically provide people a means to pursue meaningful work in their lives.

The methodology, as originally taught through Relax to the Max, focuses on providing massage that is both safe for the customer and safe for the practitioner, using techniques that minimize stress to the practitioner's body. Follow the directions of your instructor and you'll be on your way to a long, soul-satisfying career in chair massage.

Enjoy,

Eric Brown
Founder, Relax to the Max

Table of Contents

The Wonderful World of Chair Massage

Chair Massage is one of the biggest innovations in the massage industry since Swedish massage was popularized in North America over 150 years ago. Don't underestimate the power of a simple backrub in changing both the massage industry and your practice.

I take massage very seriously. For example:

- I've taught literally thousands of therapists over my career at some of the most prestigious massage therapy schools in Canada

- I've been involved in drafting the Standards of Practice for massage therapy legislation in the province of Ontario

- I was commissioned to write a research-based massage textbook by a large American publisher

- I've promoted the massage industry through appearances and interviews in national newspapers and on national television

- But, despite my efforts to "professionalize" and "medicalize" massage, I have what many of my massage therapy colleagues would consider a distasteful and objectionable obsession. If you know me even a little bit, you know that I am wildly passionate about (dare I say the word?)

- …backrubs!

- That's right! Backrubs in those specially designed massage chairs. My colleagues shake their heads in disbelief and ask themselves …

- Why Chair Massage?

I love chair massage because I believe that it has the potential to truly make massage a mainstream service - accessible to everyone.

Despite its apparent popularity, massage is still not used by the masses. Canadian census data shows that only 2% of the population has had massage in the previous year. A more recent report from the Ontario government shows that only 2½ percent of the public has had a massage in the past year.

It doesn't seem to make any sense.

You see massage in the media all the time. It seems so acceptable nowadays.

When you massage a friend's shoulders how likely are they to say, "Stop! Stop! I hate when you massage me. It feels terrible." Never in a million years because like everyone else on this planet they love massage.

We need touch to survive. That's why touch is associated with the pleasure centers in our brain. Every survival function is tied to those pleasure centers in the mid-brain – for example, sex and eating. Our nervous systems are hardwired to make sure that we get it. So we're designed to seek out touch and we enjoy it. So if people need it so badly and enjoy it so much, then why don't they get massage?

To answer that question you need to look at classical massage or Swedish massage (I'll call it table massage to differentiate it from chair massage) from the viewpoint of the customer…

Stand in their shoes and look at massage as though you know nothing. To paraphrase Palmer, to get a massage…

> "…you have to go into a small room behind closed doors, take off all your clothes and lie prone on a table while a stranger rubs greasy oil all over your body. To top it off you have to fork over a lot of money for the privilege."

I know it bothers many massage professionals to think of massage from this viewpoint, but by and large, that's the public perception of massage. And when looked at from that perspective, it seems as if the massage industry is purposely trying to discourage the average person from using massage.

A little side note: That above quote is roughly paraphrased from David Palmer, the "father of chair massage". I'm a massage therapist and when I first heard those words spoken at his workshop, I nearly packed my stuff and left the room. That's how offended I was.

You have to understand that there are many psychological blocks that prevent people from using massage on a regular basis.

For example, to get Swedish massage or table massage the client has to undress. And as a society, we're just not comfortable with nudity. According to the "1999 National Survey on Canadian Attitudes Towards Nudity" by Market Facts, less than 40% of Canadians have walked or would walk around their house nude. We are not even comfortable sleeping naked. Less than 60% of Canadians have slept or would sleep nude. Given that information, can we, as massage professionals, think that the average person will feel comfortable being naked with a complete stranger like you or me? I don't think so!

In addition, North Americans are just not a very touch intensive society. One study tracked the average number of times per hour that conversing couples touched each other in public in four different cultures. In San Juan (Puerto Rico) the number was 180 and in Paris 110. In Florida, couples only touched each other two times per hour on average. (Likely an accident while passing the ketchup.)

Couples in London scored the lowest possible. The researchers found that they didn't touch each other at all! If couples don't feel comfortable touching each other, how comfortable is the average person going to feel being touched by a complete stranger like you or me? Not very!

You really have to get out of your own brain and into the heads of your potential customers. Just because you may feel comfortable being naked and being touched in a typical massage setting doesn't mean everyone else does. That's a hard concept for most massage professionals to understand and I won't be surprised if you have your back up a little as I'm saying this.

I'm not surprised because I felt the same kind of resistance when this was first pointed out to me. I loved massage so much that it never occurred to me that other people wouldn't feel exactly the same way about it.

Why aren't massage professionals busier?

I've surveyed both the public and massage therapists on the question: Why don't people use massage?

It never fails that the average person reports that they feel uncomfortable getting undressed. On the other hand massage therapists seldom consider this an issue. In my workshops, therapists usually mention price as the biggest obstacle.

But beyond nudity there are other issues to consider.

- It's not convenient for people in a variety of ways: You have to go through the hassle of traveling to a clinic. The time it takes to travel back and forth and to actually get the massage means you've lost a big chunk of your day. And once you're covered in oils, you really can't do much until you take a shower and get cleaned up.

- People don't have the time. Time is the currency of the decade. Time is often much more valuable to people than money. Most massage sessions are an hour long– then there's the traveling time. A one-hour massage can easily take two or two and a half hours out of your day.

- There's the fear of the unknown. Massage is not visible. It's done behind closed doors so that people do not know what to expect. They don't know who's touching them or how they are going to be touched. They are afraid of the practitioner acting inappropriately.

- They are afraid that they will respond to the massage inappropriately. They are afraid of being exposed or embarrassed. There are many unknown variables to be afraid about.

- Then there are body image issues. As a massage professional, how many times do you have people apologizing about their bodies in a typical day? Your clients say things like,

"I haven't been to the gym this month." "I probably ate too much over the holidays. I'm starting a diet soon." "I hope you don't cut yourself on my legs."

- Cost can be an issue for some people, but is likely one of the smallest obstacles preventing people from getting massage.

- Then there is the perception of massage as a luxury. Because most massage professionals label themselves as "therapists," people feel that they should have something wrong with them to justify booking an appointment. In reality, most people just want to relax. Despite an industry trend to "medicalize" massage, most people simply use massage for relaxation and stress management. Look at the American Massage Therapy Association's yearly surveys. Rehabilitation has never made it into the top three reasons why people use massage.

To sum up, we have the situation where people are secretly and desperately wanting massage, but the psychological barriers to getting massage are too great to allow them to use it.

The ideal massage...

So, if we could create an ideal massage service that is able to overcome the psychological barriers, we should have a service that truly has universal appeal and that will get used by people.

And that's exactly the kind of massage service that's available through chair massage.

Chair massage removes all the barriers that prevent people from using massage:

- It's done through the clothing to save people the time and discomfort of having to get undressed and on a table

- No messy oils are used so you don't feel slimy and your clothes don't get stained?

- It is convenient because it can be brought right into a person's office or home

- Because it takes only 15 to 30 minutes, no longer than a coffee break, even the busiest person can find the time to use it

- It's inexpensive – anybody can afford it

- It can be done out in the open and that makes potential customers feel safe because they can see exactly what it's all about and who's doing it

- It targets key tension areas where people need massage – the back, neck and shoulders

- It provides the type of benefit that most people want from massage – relaxation.

- And it feels great!

It's a type of massage that appeals to the masses and not just a small segment of society. Almost everybody is a prospect for chair massage.

That's why I get so excited about chair massage. It allows us to get massage to everyone. It will appeal to office workers, construction workers, young people, older people, rich and poor people, men, women and people of all cultural backgrounds.

In fact, after I was introduced to chair massage, I got so excited that I immediately bought a chair and began doing it everywhere. Within the first few months I did massage in every conceivable environment…

- Corporations

- Tradeshows

- Music festivals

- Tanning salons

- Hotels

- Street fairs

- Hair salons

- …and even in bars

Every place I did massage was a viable market for massage. And even though no one had heard of chair massage at the time, I was accepted with open arms.

There's nothing that has as much potential as chair massage to bring massage to the masses while helping you develop a thriving business. As a small example, consider this email I got from Reflexologist Marie Leonard:

> Since I graduated last May [from Relax to the Max], I have doubled my income! I am a Reflexologist and of course must wait for clients to come and see me at my office. I have found that since I now offer chair massage, I have increased my exposure exponentially. I now have steady contracts with CIBC, Nova Scotia bank in Cochrane and Timmins, OPP and Ministry of Natural Resources. This also gives me the opportunity to educate my clients on the benefits of reflexology. All in all, I am very happy that things are working out so well. Thanks for everything.

I'm not at all surprised by her success.

I sincerely hope that you'll go through this book (or the DVDs or live training), get excited about chair massage and share your newfound skills with people who desperately need massage.

The Business of Chair Massage

Discover why chair massage has so much potential to make massage accessible to the mainstream public. This chapter looks at some of the larger concepts involved in marketing chair massage and examines some professional issues around providing this service.

An education in how to build a successful chair massage business should not be considered as an afterthought or as an option. It is an absolute necessity. You can have the best technique in the world, but if you don't know how to reach people and compel them to use your services, then nobody benefits from your skills. If you want to be successful with chair massage, you have to get familiar with the business aspects of this industry. I implore you to invest in your business and marketing education.

In any discussion of the business of massage, issues around our role or our scope of practice and regulation always arise. I have no desire to get involved in the debate around these ideological issues. Instead, I want to look at the issue strictly from a marketing standpoint.

I believe that the one commonality between all massage and bodywork professionals is that we want to see people benefit from our touch skills. And to get people to benefit from our service, we need to get them to use it. And to get people to use and benefit from our service, we need to market it in a way that will have the greatest impact on the largest number of people.

The following section, *Relaxation vs. Therapy*, is an excerpt from Lesson 7 of the BodyworkBiz *Marketing Chair Massage 101* e-course. In this excerpt, I make a case for marketing chair massage as a relaxation service (or personal care service) rather than for therapy or rehabilitative purposes.

Relaxation vs. Therapy

I don't want to delve into the issue of what a massage therapist is and how the industry should be regulated. Instead I'd like to look specifically at some arguments or opinions as it relates to chair massage.

As I've already mentioned, I have a strong bias for chair massage being strictly a relaxation service. I have French blood in my veins. It's a very physical culture. So I'd be overjoyed if we as North Americans were to become a touchy feely culture. But that isn't likely to happen soon. So for the moment I'm content to simply get more people using massage. So for me, choosing to position chair massage as relaxation massage is largely a marketing issue to help increase the public's utilization of massage.

Now I've used the words "position" or "positioning" a number of times in previous lessons, so let me explain what that means. The average consumer is bombarded by advertising messages. It is impossible for all that information to stay in anyone's head. So what we do as consumers of numerous products and services is link concepts and words with specific product brands. Typically, we have enough room in our minds to associate one idea with one product or service. That particular product is "top of mind". For example, what names do you think of when I ask you to name a Cola? A car manufacturer? A toothpaste? A watch?

Chances are the words Coke, Ford (or perhaps GM), Crest and Timex came to mind immediately. They are leaders in those categories. They have positioned themselves to be associated with those products.

Let's go a little deeper. Let's look at an everyday product like toothpaste. If you are concerned about cavities which toothpaste will you buy? Crest because "Crest fights cavities." If you want toothpaste that freshens your breath you'll buy CloseUp, so you "can get a little bit closer". If you want to remove stains from your teeth so they look their whitest, you'll buy UltraBrite. If you want toothpaste that does all three of those things, you'll buy triple protection AquaFresh. If you want all-natural, healthy toothpaste, you'll buy Tom's of Maine.

Are these toothpastes really incredibly different? Not in reality. They all have fluoride, reduce plaque, remove stains, and freshen your breath. But each of these brands has positioned itself as doing something special in the minds of the consumer. Each brand is associated with a word or concept:

Crest = Cavities

CloseUp = Fresh breath

UltraBrite = White teeth

Aquafresh = Triple protection

Tom's of Maine = Natural toothpaste

People looking for that particular benefit will gravitate towards and be faithful to that particular brand. Brands that don't have a strong position will inevitably be less successful. For example, Colgate will always take second place to Crest because it doesn't have a strong position in the consumer's mind as a cavity fighter.

Now a company like Tom's of Maine would be crazy to decide to become a cavity fighting toothpaste instead of a natural toothpaste. If they pulled their toothpaste out of health food stores and tried to get on supermarket shelves to compete with Crest as a cavity fighter, they would be doomed to a relatively quick death.

OK. Enough about toothpaste. How does this relate to chair massage? Try this little test. Ask 100 people to tell you the first word that comes into their head when they hear the word massage. What do you think the answer will be? I know what the answer will be because I've gone through this exercise many times. The results determined the name of my chair massage company.

How many do you think will say the word "therapy"? I would be surprised if more than 5% gave that answer.

Almost everyone, over 90%, will say "relaxation".

The public has placed massage in that position in their minds. To the public, massage = relaxation. Why? It doesn't really matter. What matters is that's how they see it. If you don't believe me, try the test.

Or simply look at the AMTA's consumer surveys. Two of the top three reasons for getting massage are relaxation and stress management - two sides of the same coin. The latest survey also indicated that sixty-six percent of Americans think of massage therapists as providers of a stress-reducing service outside of medicine.

This is a problem for massage therapists because once the public has positioned something in its mind, it is almost impossible to change that association. Trying to get massage positioned as "therapy" is virtually impossible. It's like Tom's of Maine beating Crest to become the consumers' choice for cavity fighting. It ain't gonna happen.

As a result, we bang our heads against the wall in frustration as we fight an entrenched public perception.

I hear this frustration from massage therapists on a regular basis. These therapists are trained in medical or rehab massage and never get to utilize their skills fully. I hear talk of the lack of respect from conventional health care workers like medical doctors and physiotherapists and even mainstream alternative professionals like chiropractors.

I hear stories of long time clients immediately going to one of these other professionals when a problem arises without the slightest consideration of consulting their massage therapist. Therapists tell me that clients dismiss their suggestions, don't follow through with adequate treatment schedules, and are not compliant with recommendations for treatment or self-care simply because they lack credibility as rehab specialists.

Despite extensive training in remedial massage by therapists in places like Ontario (2,200 hours) and British Columbia (3,000 hours), most clients simply come in for a good backrub.

It's discouraging not being able to put your skills to work in an effective way.

By positioning chair massage as a relaxation service, you are taking advantage of the position massage has in the consumer's mind and reinforcing that position, rather than fighting it and trying to destroy it. You are giving the consumer what they need, want and desire, rather than forcing a solution that they really don't care for.

In short: It makes massage easier to sell.

The bottom line: More people will use massage.

With chair massage the benefits are clear and simple. You feel better. You feel more relaxed, less tension, looser, more mobile, rejuvenated, and more alert. The benefits are immediate and real.

Furthermore, the benefits are experienced in the most powerful way: in real life, first hand, in the flesh. This will lead the consumer to an interest in more advanced forms of massage like table massage. (And when I say advanced, I'm not implying that chair massage is less valuable, but rather that table massage is a more complex service in the minds of consumers given the psychological and societal factors that we've already talked about.)

Now let's look at your own behavior as a consumer. Did your first experience with eating out take place in a fine dining establishment? When you bought your first car, was it top of the line? Your first suit? Your first stereo system? How sophisticated was your first purchase of a bottle of wine?

There is a trend in everyone's buying habits. When you buy something that you are not familiar with you tend to choose low-cost, low-risk, simple solutions first. As your experience, knowledge, and sophistication grows around that particular product or service, you move on to more expensive, complex and sophisticated versions.

My first suit was a plaid hand-me-down. My second suit was bought from a Sear's catalogue. Ah! A powder blue safari suit. I remember it fondly. (This was in the 70's of course.) My third I got from Tip Top Tailors. Now I buy rather expensive suits from brand name designers. My buying pattern is a typical consumer-buying pattern. Think back to the products and services that you use and you'll find the same pattern.

And that's exactly what will happen with people using chair massage. The average consumer is not sophisticated when it comes to bodywork. But they can understand the real benefits associated with a relaxing back or shoulder rub. As they become more knowledgeable and sophisticated, they will naturally seek out other forms of massage. It's inevitable.

To develop the massage industry we need to get as many people as possible introduced to massage in whatever form is most simple to understand and appreciate. We want to move people into the cycle of buying massage in the most accessible way possible. Consumers will then move themselves through an increasingly mature, developed and advanced buying process and will naturally make use of other forms of massage.

It's not rocket science. It's well documented human behavior.

In its simplest terms, chair massage is an entry-level service into massage for an entry-level market. In a market where the majority of people have never had a massage, this kind of accessible service is absolutely essential for the growth of the industry as a whole.

Scope of practice

As a chair massage practitioner, it is important to understand the limits of your work. This is often referred to as your *scope of practice*. If you are a regulated massage professional, this may be laid out for you in legislation.

Provided that it is legal to do, you certainly can do massage therapy or rehabilitation treatments using the massage chair. There are strong proponents for using the chair in this way – established professionals like Ralph Stevens. I think the chair provides fabulous opportunities for professionals who focus on the medical aspect of their practice. As long as they have the requisite skills, massage professionals who want to use the chair this way have my wholehearted support.

However, my bias from a marketing perspective is to see chair massage positioned primarily as a relaxation service. So the following discussion on scope of practice focuses on that particular aspect of the service.

With a short training program, like the entry-level training program I've developed at Relax to the Max, participants are trained to do relaxation or wellness massage. Any benefits, effects, or results that come about besides relaxation are simply side effects and we cannot take responsibility for achieving that result.

For example, let's say that someone with a headache wants chair massage. In your role as a provider of relaxation massage it would be inappropriate to promise that the headache will go away. You should be clear that it's not your intention to treat the headache. Your role is to help that person relax. Now, they may very likely find that the headache is gone after the session. However, you can't claim to have "fixed" that person's headache. The headache relief is simply a positive side effect of the relaxation that has been elicited.

It would be ethically wrong to claim to do therapy or rehabilitation through massage if that is not the scope of your training. You don't want to mislead the public into thinking that you are trained in this regard by calling yourself a therapist unless you have the skills to assess, diagnose and treat specific musculoskeletal conditions.

In order to be honest and clear with the public, it is vitally important that you use proper language when describing yourself or your services. You must use language that avoids confusion and that creates a distinction between rehabilitation and relaxation massage.

Consider the following terms and how they compare:

Massage therapy	Chair massage
▪ Massage therapy ▪ Medical massage	▪ Chair massage ▪ Seated massage ▪ Relaxation massage
▪ Massage therapist	▪ Massage practitioner ▪ Massage technician
▪ Treatment	▪ Session ▪ Service
▪ Patient ▪ Client	▪ Customer ▪ Client
▪ Illness	▪ Wellness
▪ Rehabilitation	▪ Prevention
▪ Massage practice	▪ Massage business

Let's look at how some of these words and concepts are defined.

The term *therapeutic* as defined by Dorland's Medical Dictionary is "that which pertains to the science and art of healing or curing." Although one could argue that a brisk walk is therapeutic in many ways, the general association the public has with the word *therapy* or *therapeutic* is medical treatment of some problem or disease. If we look at a standard dictionary (Oxford School Dictionary), the word *therapy* is defined as "remedial treatment of disease." By association, *massage therapy* is the rehabilitation of physical problems or diseases through the use of massage and a massage therapist is the paramedical professional who treats these physical problems with manual (hands on) techniques.

To avoid confusion, use the term *chair massage* or *seated massage* instead of *massage therapy*. You could also choose the terms *on-site massage*, or simply *relaxation massage*.

Because you do not do therapy, the term *massage practitioner, massage technician* or simply *massage professional* could be used. Regulatory bodies in some States actually use the term *massage technician* in legislation to describe someone who has a small amount of training and who does relaxation massage. We have chosen not to use this term simply because a tendency to use acronyms blurs the line between *massage therapists (MT)* and *massage technicians (MT)*. The term *practitioner* simply refers to someone who practices a profession. It is sometimes applied to people in the paramedical professions, but for lack of a better term, this word best describes your role with the least confusion.

A *treatment* is a "method of counteracting disease or of applying remedy for injury" (Webster's Dictionary). Thus, as a chair massage practitioner we do not do *massage treatments*. Instead, we could advertise *massage sessions* or talk about our *massage service*. Likewise, the people we massage are our *customers* or *clients* and not our *patients*. A *patient* is a person who is ill or is undergoing treatment for disease. The term *client* is sometimes used as a synonym for patient, but is commonly used in ambulatory care settings as well as other professional settings that do not necessarily involve healthcare.

Rather than working with people who are sick or ill, we most often will be working with people who are generally healthy. Instead of dealing with illness, we are helping people maintain wellness. Instead of being involved in rehabilitation, we are helping to manage stress and are therefore playing a preventative role.

Another term you should be aware of is *practice*. While the term does not always refer to a medical business, it would be better to refer to your operation simply as *a massage business* rather than a *massage practice*. This again provides clarity and helps the public understand that you are not providing a medical or paramedical service, but a personal care service.

Here's a definition of "wellness personal service massage" as outlined by Sandy Fritz in the book *Mosby's Fundamentals of Therapeutic Massage*. It's a little lengthy, but it provides a clear idea about the role of a chair massage practitioner.

Wellness personal service massage:

"A nonspecific approach to massage with a focus on the assessment procedures to determine contraindications to massage, the need for referral to other health care professionals, and the development of a health enhancing physical state for the client. The massage session plan is developed by combining information, desired results, and directions from the client with the skills of the massage practitioner to develop an individualized massage session aimed to normalization of the body systems. This normalization is achieved through external manual stimulation of the nervous, circulatory, and respiratory systems, connective tissue, and muscle to provide generalized stress reduction, a decrease in muscle tension, symptomatic relief of pain related to soft tissue dysfunction, increased circulation, and other benefits similar to exercise or other relaxation responses produced by therapeutic massage to increase the well being of the client."

To sum up, from a marketing standpoint, it makes good business sense to present chair massage as a relaxation or wellness service. Whether you decide to go that route is up to you. But in either case, it's important to communicate what you do in a clear and honest way with your customers.

And this leads us to a broader issue, that is, conducting your business with the highest ethical standards.

Code of Ethics

If you are licensed or belong to an association, you may be required to adhere to a Code of Ethics or specific Standards of Practice. Be sure you are familiar with and follow the rules and regulations that you are obliged to operate under.

If you are not covered under any such rules, it would be useful to establish a personal Code of Ethics or Business Standards that you can hold yourself to. Use these principles to guide you in making decisions about your actions. Publish these standards on your website or make them available to clients as a public display of your professionalism and as a public statement of accountability.

I've reviewed Codes of Ethics from a number of associations. Below I've listed some of the common features of these documents and worded them in a way that you can model for your own use.

Suggested standards...

SCOPE OF PRACTICE

I will provide only those services that are within the scope of my training. This includes only services that I am qualified to perform safely and competently. I will never hesitate to refer my client to an appropriately qualified professional when my client's condition requires skills beyond the scope of my training.

DISCLOSURE

I will honestly inform the client of the type and scope of my service. I will be sure that the client knows what to expect and will be sure to obtain consent to proceed with the massage as discussed.

QUALITY

I will demonstrate a commitment to provide the highest quality of service for the benefit of my clients. I will seek to improve my skills on a continuing basis.

SAFETY

I will take all appropriate measures to ensure the safety of my client. I will screen the client for conditions that would contraindicate the use of my services and take appropriate action if it is not in the client's best interest to make use of my services including refusal of services and/or referral to a qualified professional.

CONFIDENTIALITY

I will respect the confidential nature of any information that is shared with me by my client.

RESPECT

I will respect the client's right to refuse, modify, or terminate treatment regardless of any prior consent. I will avoid discrimination on the basis of race, color, gender, sexual orientation, social class, age, disability, religion or political beliefs.

PROFESSIONALISM

I will be committed to working in partnership and collaborating with other professionals for the benefit of my clients.

LEGAL OBLIGATIONS

I will seek to comply with any applicable laws or regulations that are relevant to my business and services. I will not provide services while my ability to practice is impaired by drugs or alcohol.

MAINTAIN BOUNDARIES

I will maintain appropriate boundaries with my client. I will refrain from any sexual conduct or activities with my client.

The Benefits of Massage

What does massage do? And how does it work? Although massage can have a far-reaching social impact, this chapter will focus on some of the basic physiological effects. We'll finish off by looking at how massage can counter the effects of stress.

There is a large part of the massage industry that is attempting to restore massage to its rightful place as a powerful healing art. Since the mid-80's, in particular, there has been an increasing emphasis on the medical or rehabilitative aspects of massage as a way to bring some credibility and respectability to an industry that has long been associated with the world of prostitution.

I received my training in Ontario, Canada, a province that has some of the highest training standards in the world for massage therapists. I began my training in the 80's at the beginning of this recent trend to "medicalize" massage. My colleagues and I were well trained in orthopedic assessment and received a great education in various forms of manual medicine.

And I've seen the powerful benefits of massage first hand through my career. I've had my share of success stories, both in my own clinical practice and as a clinic supervisor looking after world-class dancers at the National Ballet School and high-level varsity athletes at the University of Toronto and Ryerson University. I'm a zealous advocate for the use of massage as a rehabilitative tool. In this respect, it deserves equal standing beside chiropractic and physiotherapy. However, I can't help but believe that massage is much more than an alternative to an aspirin, ultrasound, or a spinal adjustment.

If you have been part of this industry for any length of time, you can't help but notice the transformational effect it has on people. Not just on their tissues, but in their psyche and in their souls. And although these kinds of effects are largely unintended, they are much more profound than the simple resolution of an injury or pain problem.

I think that in our attempt to gain credibility by aligning more closely with the medical industry and by focusing on the physiological aspects of massage, we've neglected a much broader role that we can play in society, mainly, being advocates for touch as a positive social value.

Western society, and this includes the medical profession, not only minimizes the importance of touch, but marginalizes touch and views it as something to be avoided. Noted touch-researcher Tiffany Field rightly refers to America as a "touch-taboo" society. There are increasing restrictions placed on touch largely due to fears around sexual harassment, physical abuse and the potentially damaging legal repercussions that could arise from what could be perceived as inappropriate touch. I've heard more than a few educators lament the fact that they are unable to do something as simple as comfort a distressed child with a hug.

But healthy touch is important. There is a strong case to be made for the incredible value of positive social touch. And although it is out of the scope of a simple techniques book like this one, there are some great resources available in this area. I would highly suggest that everyone reads Ashley Montagu's *Touching: The Human Significance of the Skin* and Tiffany Field's *Touch* to get a sense of the social significance of touch and the value of our work. Through touch we have the ability to improve body image, reduce aggressive behavior, enhance communication, improve productivity...and the list goes on.

As massage professionals, we are uniquely positioned to be powerful ambassadors for healthy touch in a touch-starved world. We have the power to affect our environments and communities in a profound way.

Back to the physical world...

Again, it's beyond the scope of this book to delve into those issues. What I'd like to do here is answer a couple of questions that I often get asked...

What does massage do? And how does it work?

The effects of massage are numerous and oftentimes complex. Sometimes even researchers are not clear on why massage works the way it does. I did a very extensive review of the research literature for a research-based textbook that I was commissioned to work on in the early 90's. I'll summarize some of the findings below. It's a brief outline of some of the beneficial effects of massage on various systems. Where appropriate, I've included a brief outline of the mechanism through which the effect occurs.

Although I've tried to keep the explanations simple, the concepts and terminology can be difficult to understand, especially if you don't have a background in physiology. For the purposes of simple relaxation massage, it is not necessary to know these effects or the mechanism behind them. However, this information will deepen your understanding for what you do, enhance your appreciation for the value of your work and enable you to answer some of the many questions your customers will throw at you.

What's most important, always, is that your customer enjoys your touch, feels relaxed, and has an enhanced sense of wellbeing after your massage. The effects that are listed below are not things we are intentionally trying to achieve with the customer. They are simply positive side effects of your seated massage.

Muscle tone

Massage decreases muscle tension (excessive muscle tone). It does this in several ways. Firstly, by mechanically stretching the muscle fibers (or cells). Secondly, through neural reflexes that are initiated with stimulation of sensory receptors in the muscles. And lastly, through a generalized relaxation response that causes a general decrease in muscle tone.

Massage does not decrease normal muscle tone. Neither does it increase tone.

Blood flow

Massage does not increase blood flow to muscles. This is very well documented by research.

An exception to this is the percussion techniques. If these techniques are used for any length of time they will cause a short sustained increase in blood flow to the muscles. This is likely due to the traumatic nature of the technique that may cause the release of histamine or other vasodilating chemicals (substances that cause blood vessels to relax).

Massage will, however, normalize blood flow in tense muscles. When a muscle is tense it essentially squeezes off its blood supply and the muscle becomes ischemic (doesn't have enough blood). So when you decrease tension in a muscle, the blood flow can return to a normal level.

Massage does not increase overall blood flow through the body (cardiac output).

The body has homeostatic mechanisms that maintain a needed volume of blood through the tissues and a needed level of blood pressure. Any attempts to change this are countered by various reactions of the body.

While general circulation and circulation to the muscles does not increase, circulation to the skin does. Because the skin regulates body temperature by allowing more or less blood to the surface, the blood vessels in the skin are a little more dynamic. Stimulation of the skin will often cause an increase in blood flow. You can often see the person's skin turn red (called hyperemia). The redness (blood flow) will subside slowly after you stop massaging the area.

Lymph flow

Lymph is fluid that is pulled out of the tissues. It contains cellular debris and bacteria. It flows through its own system of vessels. It's usually regarded as the sewer system for the body's tissues.

Massage increases the production and flow of lymph. The flow of lymph has very little dynamic control. It is simply pushed along its route by mechanical pressure and muscle contraction. Lymph vessels, like veins, have valves that only allow the flow of fluid in one direction, toward the heart. So massage does not have to be performed towards the heart. Any compression or kneading action will move the lymph forward in the proper direction.

Fascia

Fascia is the fibrous connective tissue that surrounds all muscles. When a muscle is tense or held in a shortened position for a prolonged time, this connective tissue shortens. This can restrict your flexibility and range of motion.

The fascia is not elastic. It is more of a woven type of structure. When sufficient pressure is applied to the soft tissues, the fascia can be stretched. This stretching is essentially a tearing of the bonds between the protein strands that are woven together.

In stretching fascia, you are to a certain extent traumatizing the tissues. This is not a bad thing. The trauma occurs on a microscopic level.

The next day, the customer may feel some stiffness in their muscles. This is similar to the feeling you get when you exercise after being inactive for a while. It is called "delayed onset muscle soreness". The customer feels fine during the massage and it takes awhile for the small levels of inflammation in the muscle to develop. The stiffness typically subsides within a day or two.

The immune system

Typically massage has been shown to increase various indicators of immune function. There have been a small number of studies that have examined this issue. The mechanisms behind this effect are not fully understood.

The nervous system

The area where massage has the greatest impact is on the nervous system. The skin, from a neurological viewpoint, is tightly associated with the central nervous system (brain and spinal cord). They both come from the same embryonic tissues.

It is not exactly clear how massage affects the nervous system. In studies it has shown effects as diverse as increased weight gain in premature infants, improvements in immune function, the ability to do math computations faster and with more accuracy, decreases in aggression, improved body image and decreased levels of anxiety.

Massage, through the stimulation of proprioceptors (sensory nerves that give signals about your posture and movement), can help improve body awareness and improve posture.

Of course, one of the most notable effects on the nervous system is relaxation. With massage, a relaxation response is triggered which causes generalized decreases in muscle tone, decreased production of stress hormones, changes in the autonomic nervous system (which controls involuntary and visceral functions) moving towards restorative and regenerative processes, as well as changes in brain wave activity.

Pain

Massage is shown to have a positive impact on pain. Many of the effects on pain are likely due to the normalizing effect on muscle tension and circulation.

Massage also creates an analgesic (pain killing) effect through stimulation of the nervous system. The mechanism responsible is usually referred to as a *counter-irritant effect*. In essence, when you stimulate the skin and muscles, there is a rapid barrage of sensory signals that are sent to the spinal cord. These sensory signals override the slower moving pain signals and in a sense close their gate into the spinal cord. The analgesic effect of massage can last for minutes or it can last for days after the massage.

Stress, relaxation & the role of massage

Because relaxation is such an important element of our work, it's important that we understand a little about stress and relaxation, and in particular how we can best structure our massage to achieve a relaxation response.

I'll give a quick summary here. For more details on these issues refer to Appendix XXX which will provide a much broader understanding of this complex topic.

Stress is a physical response. It is elicited in response to anything that is perceived as a threat, that is, anything that carries potential for harm.

The things that elicit stress are referred to as stressors. What's common to all stressors is that they involve change: good or bad, internal or external, minor (hassles) or major (life changes). Change is interrelated with uncertainly, unpredictability and ambiguity.

We mostly hear about stress in the context of emotional stress. However, any stimulus, including tactile, auditory, and visual stimuli can initiate the response. For example, if you are sitting quietly with your eyes closed and you suddenly feel someone touching your leg, that new sensation immediately causes your nervous system to be stimulated and initiate a stereotypical stress response.

The response to any stressor can be modified by your appraisal of the stimulus. In the appraisal of a new stimulus, your mind weighs the possibility of harm. In the above example, if you were sitting on a patio relaxing with your mate, then the touch would not be stressful, simply because you know it's harmless.

One of the key factors involved in the appraisal of potential harm is your level of control over the stressor. In an emotional context, your level of control is determined by the gap between the demand placed upon you and the resources you have to deal with that demand. Uncertainty, unpredictability, and ambiguity in any situation lower your perceived control. If the stimulus is threatening, or the demands exceed your ability to adapt, a stress response is elicited.

The stress response is a complex pattern of hormonal, neurological, and musculoskeletal changes. Its entire purpose is to prepare the body for action – "fight or flight". The body seeks to avoid or remove the stimulus.

I think it is important to note that stress is a response that is entirely geared toward preparing your body for physical action. Every physiological change that occurs during a stress response, whether it is hormonal or neurological, is for the sole purpose of preparing for muscular activity.

You can see that various steps are involved in creating a stress response. This is referred to as the *stress pathway*. A stressor > leads to an appraisal of the stressor > leads to the stress response.

Our first goal in performing a massage is to help the customer avoid or minimize any possible stress response. Since change is a key component of every stressor, every aspect of your behavior and the massage should, to the fullest extent possible, be certain, predictable, and unambiguous.

Examples of these traits in your behavior include:

- Setting realistic expectations of the massage

- Communicating a clear outline of your massage procedure and clear instructions for customers

- Getting consent from the customer and giving them control to modify, change, or stop their massage for any reason

- Being upfront with policies and procedures

- Being clear on what they are to do after the massage is finished

Examples of these traits in the actual massage include:

- Repeating techniques or sets of techniques

- Using a consistent system for applying the techniques

- Consistency in approach, pressure, sequencing, transitions, etc.

- Using a massage routine that is repeated for each visit

Our second goal in performing massage is to elicit a relaxation response. Its elicitation is similar to the stress response. Just as there is a stress pathway (stressor > appraisal > stress response), there is also a relaxation pathway: relaxor > appraisal > relaxation response.

The relaxor (relaxation stimulus) does not demand change. For example, a mantra in meditation involves repetition of a benign phrase. In the case of massage, the relaxor is tactile stimulation (touch).

In the appraisal process, there must be potential for benefit or at the very least, the stimulus must be benign.

Based on this appraisal, a relaxation response is elicited. The relaxation response is essentially the opposite of the stress response. It promotes various restorative processes and is often referred to as a "rest and digest" response. Rather than fighting the stimulus or fleeing, the body seeks to orient itself towards the stimulus and assimilate it in some way.

Most researchers agree that there are several conditions required for relaxation to occur. These include:

1. Safety

2. Pleasure

3. Restriction of environmental stimuli

In addition, there are cognitive or mental skills that may enhance a person's ability to relax. The stronger these skills are, the more the person will be able to benefit from relaxation. These skills include:

1. Focusing: the ability to identify, differentiate, maintain attention on, and return attention to simple stimuli for extended periods of time

2. Passivity: the ability to stop unnecessary goal-directed and analytic activity

3. Receptivity: the ability to tolerate and accept experiences that may be uncertain, unfamiliar, or paradoxical

Because relaxation has received so little study, we don't really know how it works, that is, the mechanisms involved in its elicitation. I've come across several plausible mechanisms of relaxation:

1. Cognitive diversion: This theory states that a benign stimulus, like tactile stimulation that occurs with massage, diverts the mind's attention. Instead, of focusing on potentially stressful thoughts, the mind is "forced" to focus on the new and harmless sensations. As a result, physiological responses to the stressful thoughts slowly subside. The theory is sound, but it fails to really get at the underlying mechanisms of relaxation.

2. Psycho-physiological principle: Behind this mechanism is the belief that every emotional state is inextricably linked with a related pattern of musculoskeletal activity. Because of the sensation you feel in your body, an emotional state is triggered and vice versa. For example, if you feel happy, your face responds by smiling. Conversely, if you are smiling, your mind responds by feeling happy. Massage, through both direct and reflex mechanisms, causes the muscles to relax and this removes the physical foundation for the emotion of stress.

3. Release of anti-stress hormones: Tactile stimulation may mediate the release of various anti-stress hormones. One example is the hormone oxytocin, which has been referred to in the popular press as the "love hormone" or the "cuddle chemical." There is a great deal of data in the research literature that associates various types of tactile stimulation with increases in oxytocin levels.

Overall, we don't know a lot about relaxation. Our understanding of relaxation parallels our understanding of stress 50 years ago. There's much to be discovered. But even though we don't understand exactly what relaxation is and how it's produced, there is undeniable evidence that reducing stress and encouraging relaxation has tremendous health benefits. And massage can play a vital role in this regard.

Anatomy

*It's important to be familiar with the structures that you'll be massaging.
We'll cover some basic terminology that will help us discuss these
structures. We'll also look at some of the basic musculoskeletal
structures and then examine the muscles that we'll be massaging in more
detail.*

In this book, we will be looking primarily at the structure of the body – the anatomy. Little
attention will be given to the way it works (physiology), or the things that can go wrong with it
(pathology).

This is by no means a comprehensive explanation of the structures you will be massaging. It's
more of a sketch. If you have little training in anatomy, this will improve your understanding of
all that stuff you're feeling under the skin and enhance your hands-on skills.

You'll notice that the illustrations are somewhat schematic and often represent the tactile
experience of these structures rather than the anatomic reality.

General anatomic terminology

To discuss the structure of the body, it's important that a language or terminology is used that everybody can understand. This allows us to describe the body in an accurate way so that everybody has a clear idea of what's being said.

To aid the communication process, we will look at several sets of terminology:

1. Directional terminology: Used to describe where structures are relative to each other.
2. Anatomic regions: Used to outline the general areas where structures are located.
3. Movement terminology: Used to describe the direction of movement at the various joints.
4. Anatomic structures: The specific names of various bones, joints, and muscles.

Directional terminology

To describe where various structures are relative to each other we will assume that the body is in what is commonly called **anatomical position**. In anatomical position a person is standing upright, facing forward with the hands down by the sides. The palms are forward and the fingers are pointing to the ground. All references to the position of structures will assume the person is in this position unless otherwise indicated.

We always describe the location of one structure relative to a reference point or **landmark**. For example, you would not say, "My forehead is superior." Instead you would say, "My forehead is superior to my nose." In this case your nose is the landmark. The landmark does not have to be a specific structure. It can be a region. For example, the forearm is distal to the upper arm or the pectoral (chest) region is anterior to the thoracic spine.

The terms are paired. Each has an opposite. For example, if we say that something is *superior*, it implies that there is another structure that is *inferior*.

The attached illustration outlines the directional terminology that we will be using. In particular, be familiar with these terms that we will use most frequently in class:

- medial/lateral
- superior/inferior
- anterior/posterior
- proximal/distal

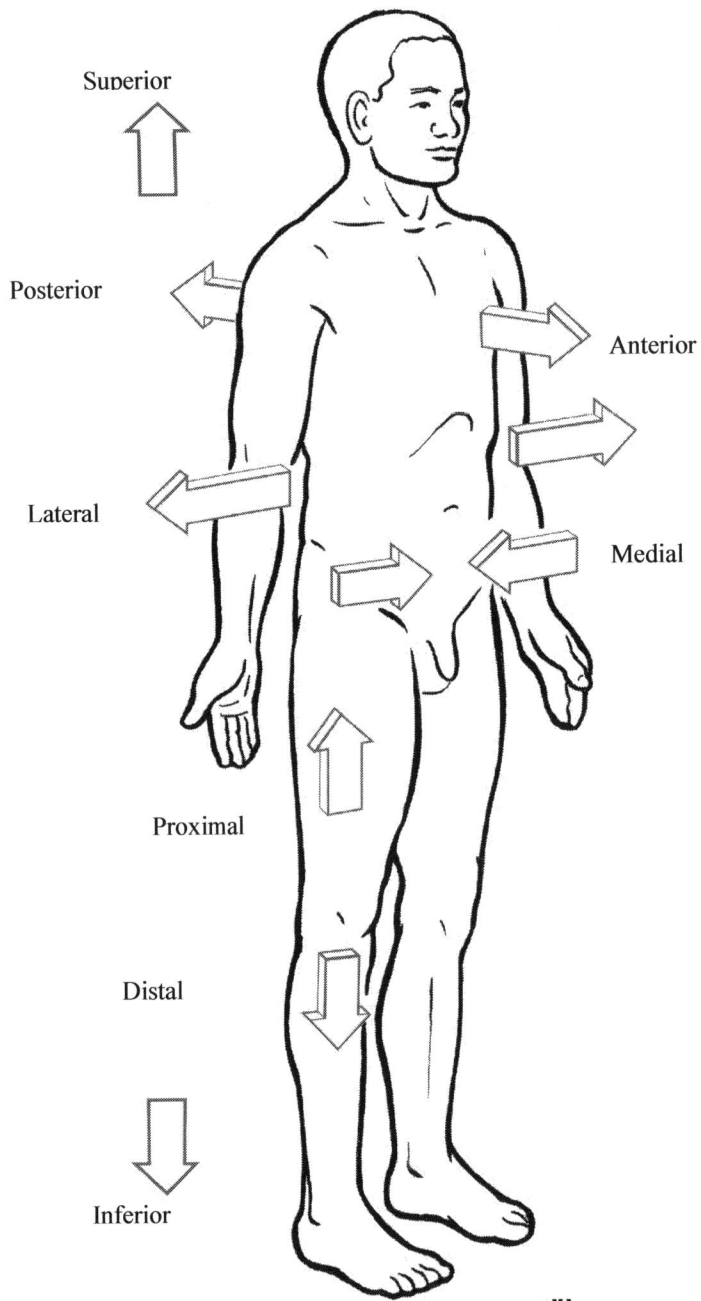

Superior

Posterior

Anterior

Lateral

Medial

Proximal

Distal

Inferior

Anatomic regions

We will often use terms that describe broad anatomical regions. The regions that will be most relevant to you in doing seated massage are outlined below.

- Occipital: the back of the skull.

- Temporal: the temples at the side of the head.

- Cervical: the neck.

- Thoracic: the mid-back.

- Lumbar: the low back.

- Sacral: the area below the lumbar vertebrae at the back of the hips.

- Gluteal: the buttock area.

- Pectoral: the chest.

- Palmer: the palm of the hand.

- Plantar: the bottom of the foot.

- Dorsal: the back or top of the hand and foot

Movement terminology

There are specific terms used to accurately describe the movements that happen at the various joints in the body. Below is a list of these terms and a brief explanation.

- Elevation: to lift, or raise part of body, for example, shrugging the shoulders.

- Depression: to lower a part of the body, for example, pushing the shoulders down.

- Protraction: to move a part of the body forward, for example, rounding the shoulders forward.

- Retraction: to move a part of the body backward, for example, pulling the shoulders back.

- Flexion: decrease the angle of a joint, for example, bending the elbow.

- Extension: increase the angle of a joint, for example, straightening the elbow.

- Lateral bending or side flexion: bending the vertebral column to the right or left side.

- Abduction: to move a body part away from the center/mid-line of the body, for example, lifting your arm up to the side.

- Adduction: to move a part of the body towards the center/mid-line of the body, for example, bringing your arm across your body.

- Rotation: revolve a part around a longitudinal axis.

- Internal rotation: to rotate towards the center/mid-line of the body, for example, rotating your leg so that your toes point inward.

- External rotation: to rotate away from the center/mid-line of the body, for example, rotating your leg so that your toes point outward.

- Circumduction: combination of many movements allowing part to move in a large circle, for example, swinging your arm in a large circle.

- Pronation: to move the palm down. This term can also be applied to the foot.

- Supination: to move the palm up. This term can also be applied to the foot.

Although these terms describe movement, they are sometimes used to refer to a static position relative to anatomical position. So, for example, if someone is standing with their elbow bent we say that the elbow is in flexion.

The table below outlines some major joints and the movements that can occur at these joints:

Joint	Action
Intervertebral joints (where two vertebra meet; all regions of the spine)	Flexion, extension, lateral flexion, rotation
Shoulder (also called the glenohumeral joint)	Flexion, extension, abduction, adduction, internal and external rotation, circumduction
Elbow	Flexion, extension
Forearm (consists of two joints: the proximal and distal radioulnar joints)	Supination, pronation
Wrist	Flexion, extension, abduction, adduction
Knuckles (metacarpophalangeal joints)	Flexion, extension, abduction, adduction
Fingers (interphalangeal joints)	Flexion, extension
Hip	Flexion, extension, abduction, adduction, internal and external rotation, circumduction
Knee	Flexion, extension

Movement terminology

Here are the types of movement that occur in the body. (E = Extension, F = Flexion)

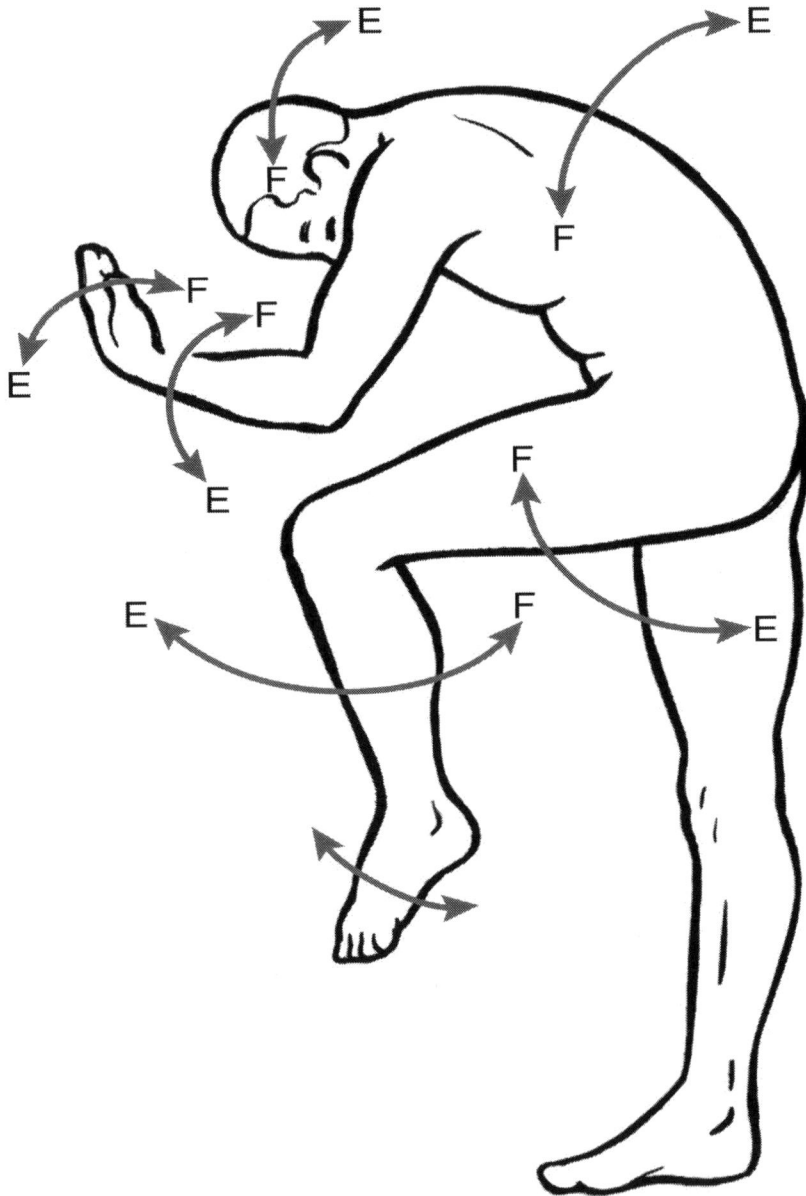

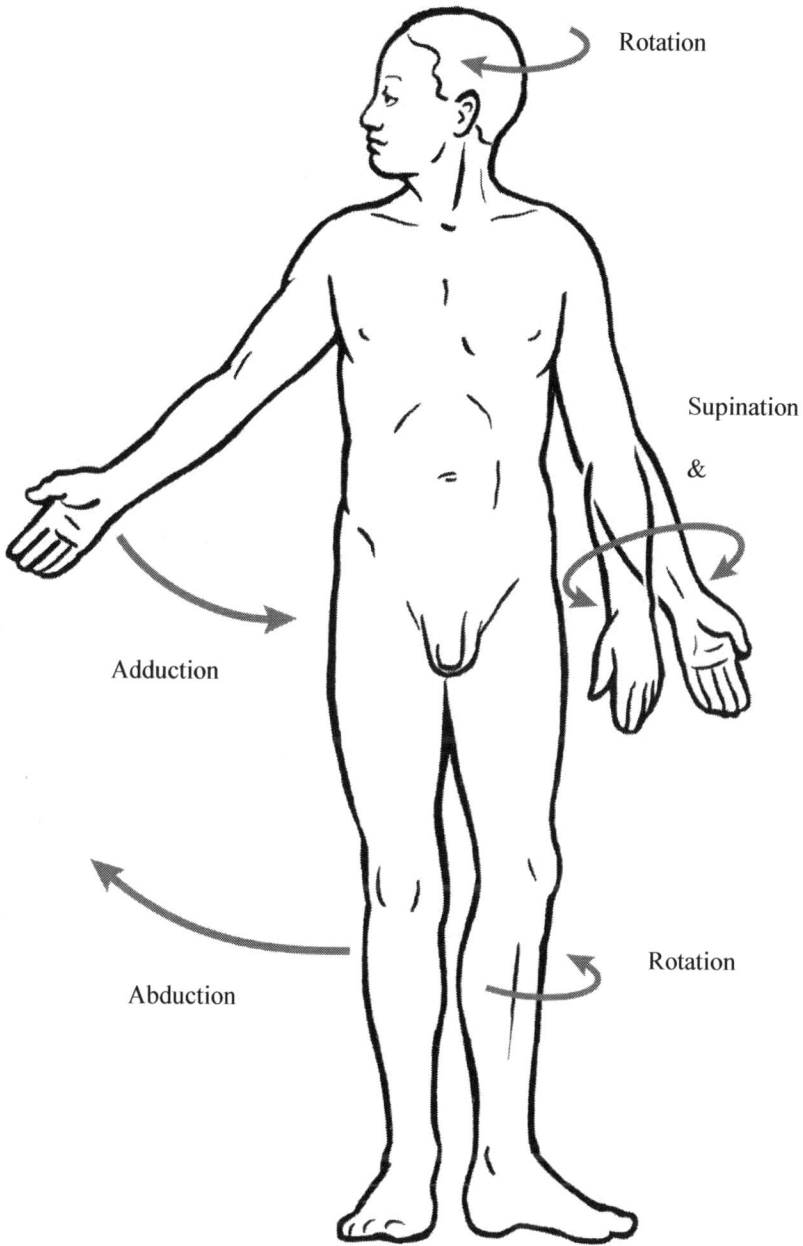

Rotation

Supination

&

Adduction

Abduction

Rotation

Basic anatomical structures – a summary

Bones

We often think of bones as lifeless material that sits in our bodies. In fact, bone is a living tissue that is filled with cells that are metabolically active. Bone consists of a framework of connective tissue that is filled with calcium. It is the calcium that is stored throughout the framework that makes bones solid.

Bone has a variety of functions:

It **provides a framework** for the body. It gives the body its characteristic shape and posture.

It **stores minerals** that the body needs to function. We know that bones contain calcium, but they also hold many other minerals including potassium, sodium, magnesium, sulfur, and copper. As the body needs these minerals, they are pulled out of the bone. If you have excess of these minerals, they are stored in the bone until needed. When too much calcium is pulled out of the bones for use by the body, the bones become weak and may become deformed or break. This condition is called *osteoporosis*.

It serves as an **anchor point for muscle attachments**. To make movement happen, muscles must attach themselves to bones.

Protection of internal organs in our chest is provided by the rib cage. Protection of our brain is provide by the skull bones.

Blood is produced in bone marrow, which is located deep in bones.

There are 206 bones in the human body. The names of the bones that we will need to be familiar with can be found on the accompanying illustrations. It is important that you are familiar with the scientific names for the bones and the common names known to the layperson. For example, the bone we know as the shoulder blade would be more correctly referred to as the scapula and the collarbone is called the clavicle.

In addition, every bump, groove, hole, and edge of each bone has a name. Obviously, there are hundreds of these landmarks that could be described. We will not discuss them here, but the relevant ones will be mentioned in class. Here are a few general terms that describe some of these landmarks:

Crest: the ridge of a large bone.

Epicondyle: a small raised area at the proximal ends of the femur and humerus.

Fossa: round, shallow, cup-like depression.

Groove: a long, shallow, depression or trough.

Head: A hammerhead like protrusion that is usually round and smooth.

Tuberosity: a large, bulb-like protrusion.

Key bony structures

Bones of the back and shoulder girdle

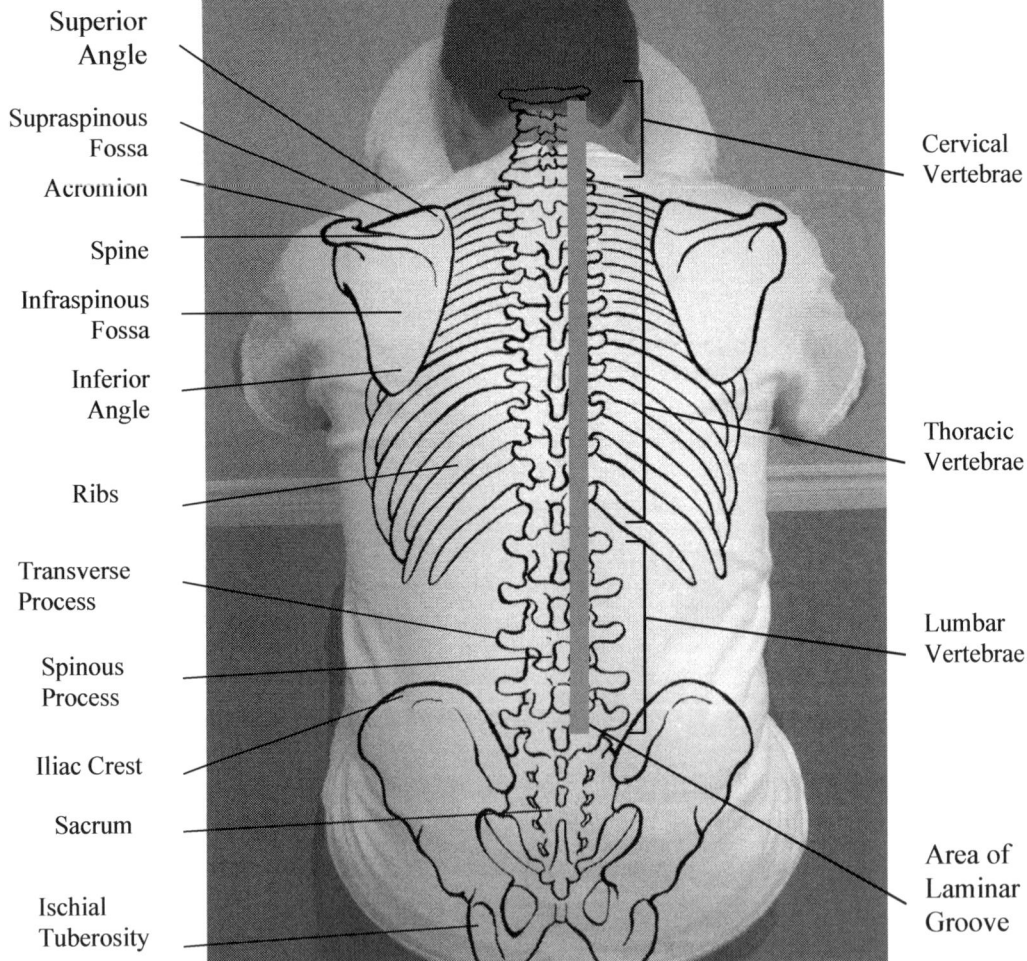

Scapula:

Superior Angle

Supraspinous Fossa

Acromion

Spine

Infraspinous Fossa

Inferior Angle

Ribs

Transverse Process

Spinous Process

Iliac Crest

Sacrum

Ischial Tuberosity

Cervical Vertebrae

Thoracic Vertebrae

Lumbar Vertebrae

Area of Laminar Groove

Bones of the arm and hand

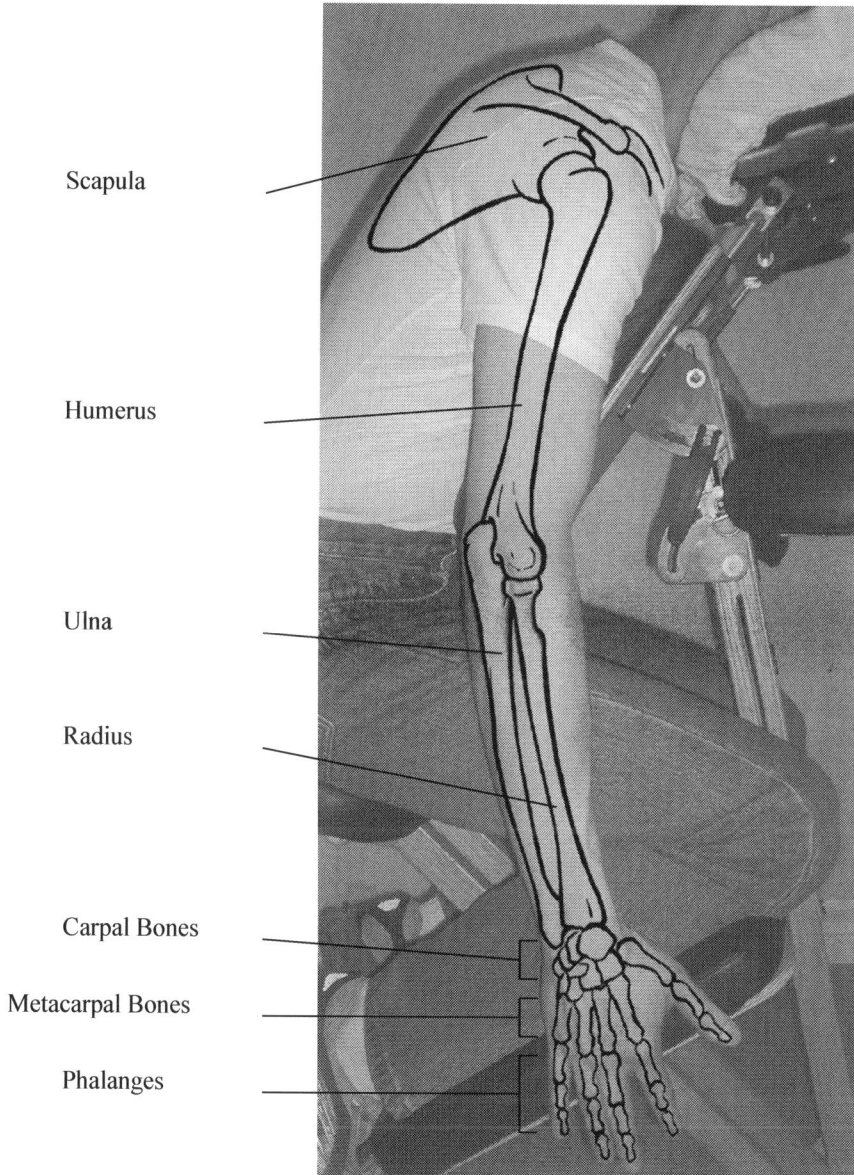

Scapula

Humerus

Ulna

Radius

Carpal Bones

Metacarpal Bones

Phalanges

Bones of the lower body

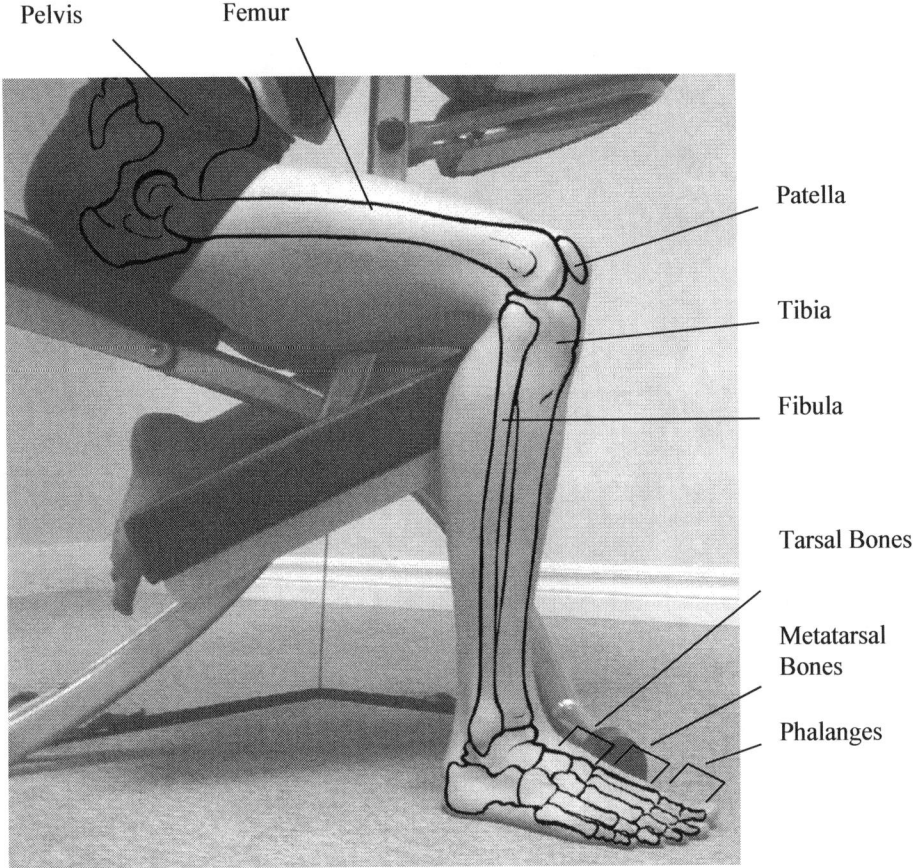

Pelvis

Femur

Patella

Tibia

Fibula

Tarsal Bones

Metatarsal Bones

Phalanges

Joints

Wherever two bones meet, a joint exists. Movement can't occur in the middle of a solid bone. Movement only happens at joints. However, movement doesn't happen at every joint. Some joints are immovable. For example, the bones of the skull come together and ossify as you grow to become rigid and immovable. Other joints allow for limited movement, like the symphysis pubis, which is a joint located at the front of the pelvis where the two pelvic bones meet.

Freely movable joints are called **synovial joints** and they are the most common type of joint in the body. There are six different types of synovial joints and each one is capable of different types of movement. For example, the hip joint is called a *ball and socket joint* and it is capable of movement in every direction. The elbow joint on the other hand is a *hinge joint* and it can only open and close (flex and extend).

Look at the accompanying illustration for a schematic look at a typical synovial joint. You can see of course that the ends of two bones are meeting one another. On the end of each bone is **cartilage**. Cartilage is a smooth, spongy material. It acts as a shock absorber and allows the bones to glide smoothly against one another.

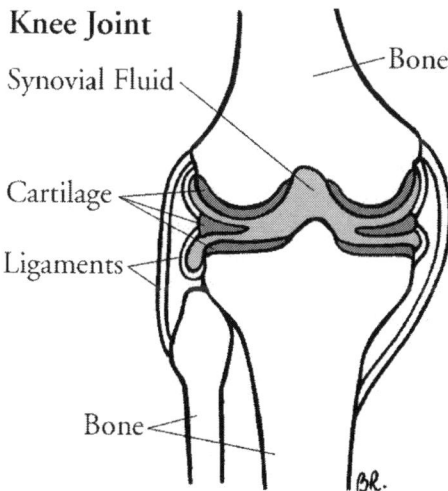

Knee Joint

Synovial Fluid

Bone

Cartilage

Ligaments

Bone

BR.

There is a fibrous material (connective tissue) that covers the bones that is called *periosteum*. When this fibrous material reaches the end of the bone it continues across to the other bone. It thus forms a sleeve over the joint that encapsulates the joint. The fibrous material that crosses over the joint is called the *joint capsule*. Within this capsule is a special lubricating fluid called *synovial fluid*.

To provide support to the joint so that the bones don't slip off one another, the capsule thickens where needed and strong fibrous cords are formed. These fibrous structures are **ligaments**. So the function of a ligament is to attach one bone to another bone.

Ligaments often determine what movement can happen at a joint. For example, at the elbow joint there are strong ligaments on the medial and lateral sides. If you hold your arm in anatomical position, you'll see that you can't move your lower arm away from your side by moving your elbow joint. The ligaments prevent this movement. If it moves away it's because you're making the movement happen from your shoulder joint and you can see in this case that your elbow remains in a straight, locked position. You can however, move your forearm towards your upper arm and return it to the anatomical position. There are no ligaments on the front or back of your elbow that prevent this flexion and extension movement.

The joints that will be particularly relevant for the purposes of this book are listed in the table located in the *Movement Terminology* section above. This table also includes a list of movements that occur at the joint.

Muscles

It should be noted that there are several types of muscles. Although they essentially function in the same way, each type has a modification in structure that helps it perform its function better. *Cardiac muscle* is a special type of muscle that is found only in the heart. *Smooth muscle* is found in organs, glands and blood vessels. For example, the muscles in your intestine that move food along are smooth muscles. The type of muscle that we are referring to when we talk about movement of the body is called **skeletal muscle**.

Muscle

Tendon

Bone

Muscles, like bones, are wrapped in a fibrous tissue. This fibrous tissue around the muscles is called **fascia**. Fascia holds muscle fibers together and is responsible for the shape of each individual muscle. When the fascia reaches the end of the muscle fibers it continues off the end and attaches itself by literally weaving itself into the fibrous tissue of a bone (the periosteum). This fibrous tissue thickens as it comes off the muscle and attaches to a bone so that it forms a strong link to the bone that can withstand strong pulling forces of the muscle. This fibrous band that connects a muscle to a bone is called a **tendon**.

Muscles provide the force for movement. Every muscle has at least two points of attachment on the bones. These attachment points are usually referred to as the *origin* and *insertion*. The origin is typically the most proximal attachment for the tendon at one end of the muscle and the insertion is the distal attachment for the tendon on the other end. Note that all muscles cross a joint otherwise they would be unable to cause movement to occur. The only exception to this is the muscles of the face that cause various facial expressions and some of the pelvic muscles. Some muscles cross more than one joint and cause movement to happen at two or more places.

What makes muscle special is its ability to contract or shorten when stimulated by a nerve impulse. Because muscles shorten, they can only pull a bone; they can't push a bone. This is a difficult concept for some people to understand because when you push a door open for example, it seems as though the muscles are pushing the arm open. In fact, in this case, muscles on the back of the arm are pulling the back edges of the bones together. Just as the muscles in the front of the arm pull the bones into a bent or flexed position, the muscles on the back of the arm pull the bones into a straight or extended position.

There are literally hundreds of different muscles in your body. We will look at just some of the muscles that we will be working on as we do seated massage. Most of the muscles described below are muscles that we can **palpate** or feel. In class we examine these muscles and learn how to identify each one. In preparation for practical classes, it is important that you memorize the names of these muscles and have a general understanding of where they are located. This overview outlines some basic information about the muscles. Be sure to refer to the accompanying illustrations.

Key anatomical structures

Palpation: Learning to Identify Muscles through Touch

Effective palpation of muscle (identification by touch) is an essential skill. It takes lots of practice along with conscious focus on what your fingers are "seeing" to develop the ability to accurately identify the muscles on which you're working. Here are some guidelines that will help you hone this skill:

- Press firmly. You need to press deeply enough to get to the levels that you want to feel.

- Move the skin with your fingers as you feel your way around. If you slide over the skin, you are not palpating firmly enough.

- Don't rush through the movement. Take your time to really focus on what your hands are feeling.

- If you are palpating something that is long, like the erector spinae muscles that run the length of the back, move your fingers back and forth at right angles (perpendicular) to the structure. That way you'll bump into or fall off the structure and get a better sense of where the edges are located.

- If you are palpating something bumpy, like the medial epicondyle (the bony bump on the inside of the elbow), do large circular movements around the area, as much as the skin will allow you to move. Again, this gives you a better sense of the shape and structure of that part.

- Distinct fleshy areas, like the upper trapezius, are best palpated with a "pincer palpation. " Use your thumb and fingers like a lobster claw and grasp the edges of the structure to determine the muscles size, shape and contours.

- **Recommended resource:** *Trail Guide to the Body: How to Locate Muscles, Bones & More* by Andrew R Biel

Muscles of the upper body

Spinal support muscles

The first group of muscles we'll look at are muscles that support the back. Although these muscles cause a wide range of movements, they work primarily as extensors, that is, they help to extend the back. If you are stooped forward (flexed forward), they will work to bring you to an upright position. If you are standing upright, they will pull your spine into a backward arch. Since most of us tend to slouch, these muscles are constantly working against gravity to stop us from falling forward. It's no wonder that these muscles get tense and tired.

ERECTOR SPINAE

The Erector Spinae are actually a group of three muscles. These long muscles run up and down the back and on either side of the spine. They help keep our spine erect, thus the name. When looking at someone's back, you will notice that there is a small mound of muscle on each side of the spine. These mounds are very prominent in the low back and they become smaller as they run up the midback and neck. The three muscles are:

Spinalis which runs up and down the back next to the spine.

Longissimus which as the name implies is a long muscle running from the top of the hips to the base of the skull.

Iliocostalis, the outermost of the three, which also attaches to the ribs.

SMALL PARASPINAL MUSCLES

These small muscles are right on top of the spine in a space called the **laminar groove** between the spinous processes and the transverse processes. These muscles are short usually the length of one to four vertebrae. Because they are small they don't have much of a role in extending the spine. Instead, they control fine movements of your back and help stabilize your vertebrae.

These muscles are difficult to feel. However, if you feel the spinous process with your fingers and then let your fingers drop off to the side of them, you will drop into the **laminar groove** and your fingers will be right on top of these small muscles.

QUADRATUS LUMBORUM

This muscle is usually referred to simply as QL by professionals. It is a square muscle (quadratus) in the low back or lumbar area (lumborum). It is a deep muscle that lies underneath the erector spinae muscles in the low back. Only the outside edge can be felt. It attaches to the lower ribs, the lumbar vertebrae and the top of the hips. It provides a lot of support for the low back. If you sit for long periods of time or have poor posture, this muscle can become quite tender.

SPLENIUS CERVICIS AND CAPITIS

These are two extensor muscles that run from the mid-back to the base of the skull. They are difficult to identify through touch simply because they are relatively deep. These muscles, especially the capitis, are referred to as "bandage" muscles because they cover and hold down the deeper neck muscles.

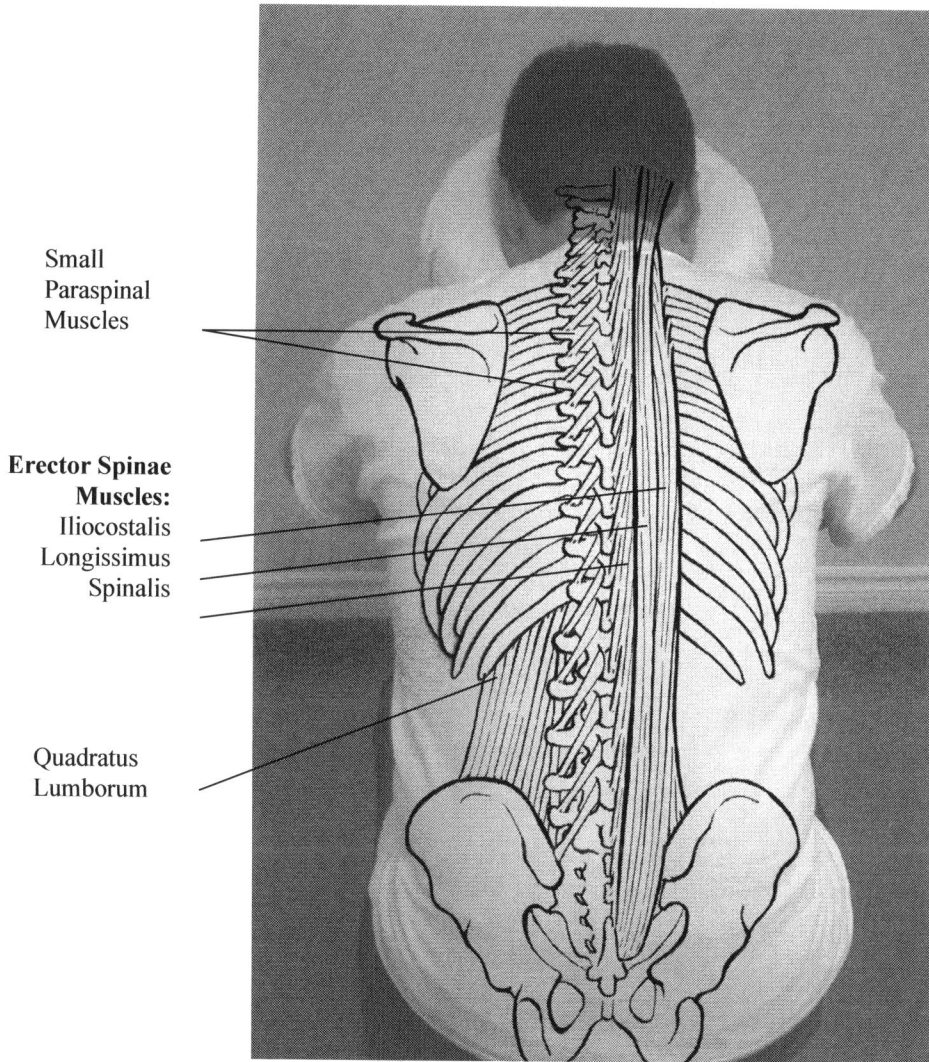

Small
Paraspinal
Muscles

Erector Spinae
Muscles:
Iliocostalis
Longissimus
Spinalis

Quadratus
Lumborum

Neck and mid-back muscles

TRAPEZIUS

This is a large muscle that covers most of the neck and mid-back. It is superficial and lies just below the skin. It looks like a large kite on your back. It is a trapezoid shape thus the name *trapezius*. It is often referred to simply as *the traps*. This is easy to remember because this is the shoulder muscle where most people "trap" their tension. Because it is so large it is usually divided into three parts: the upper traps, the middle traps, and the lower traps.

The upper traps are what people usually think of as their shoulder muscles. They are the bunches of muscle on each side of the neck that you can easily squeeze. They often get tender or painful when you are under a lot of stress. The upper traps attach onto the base of the skull and run down the neck to attach on the outer part of the collar bone (or clavicle) and part of the scapula (the spine of the scapula).

When the upper traps contract they raise the shoulders pulling them toward the ears. Conversely if only one side contracts, your head will tilt to the side.

In a static standing or sitting position, the upper traps work to hold the head upright. Most of the weight of the head falls in front of the spine so this muscle is at a disadvantage and has to work constantly to stop your head from falling forward.

The middle traps are the parts of the muscle that lie between the shoulder blade and the spine. When they contract, they pull your shoulders back. Because we tend to slouch, these muscle work hard and develop a lot of tension.

The lower traps pull your shoulder blades back and down. This part of the muscle runs from your shoulder blades to the upper part of your lumbar spine.

RHOMBOIDS

The rhomboids are similar to your mid-traps in many respects. They also attach the shoulder blades to the spine. They assist the mid-traps in retracting the shoulder blades (pulling them back). They take a great deal of punishment when we slouch as they try to prevent our shoulders from rounding forward.

LEVATOR SCAPULA

This muscle runs from the top corner of the scapular (the superior angle) and runs up the neck to attach to the sides of the neck vertebrae. It assists your upper traps in keeping your head from falling forward. It also lifts your shoulders or elevates (like an elevator) the scapula, thus the name. When you hold a phone receiver between your ear and your shoulder, the levator scapula muscle is contracting very strongly and will no doubt start to complain after a while.

As the muscle runs from the shoulder blade to the neck it twists. So it feels like a very distinct tight rope. It's difficult to feel the lower portion because it sits underneath the bulky trapezius. It is very easy to feel where it comes out from underneath the traps at the side of the neck.

SUBOCCIPITAL MUSCLES

These are small muscles that run from the neck to the skull. They are located underneath the back of the skull (called the occipital bone) and are very deep. They control fine movement of the head on the neck. Like all muscles, they are prone to becoming tense when they are held in the same position for any length of time.

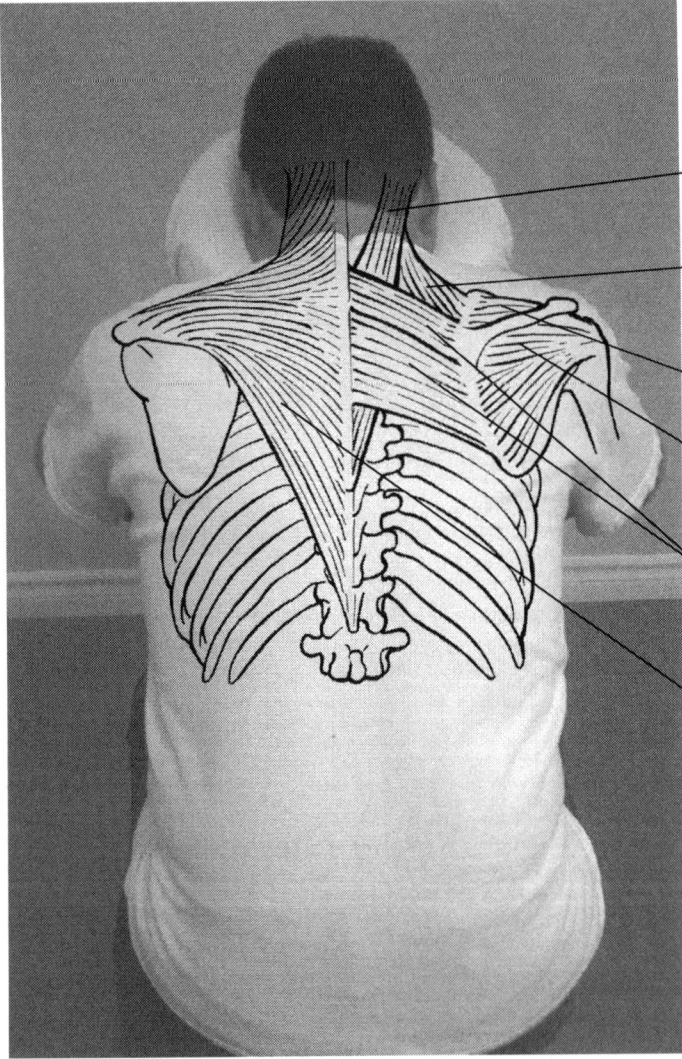

Splenius
Capitus

Levator
Scapula

Supraspinatus

Infraspinatus

Rhomboid
Major & Minor

Trapezius

58

Muscles around the shoulder

PECTORALIS MAJOR

This is your chest muscle. It is a big muscle that runs from your breastbone, ribs, and collar bone and crosses the shoulder joint to attach on the inside of the upper arm bone (the humerus). The pectoralis major tends to become short and tight simply because we have a tendency to round our shoulders. This muscle, along with the pectoralis minor described below, are commonly referred to simply as the "pecs".

PECTORALIS MINOR

This is a small chest muscle that is buried below the pectoralis major. It is difficult to feel and is usually tender. Like the pectoralis major it has a tendency to become short and tight. Although you won't be directly massaging this muscle, you will learn specific stretches for the pecs and will learn how to apply these stretches to the person in the chair.

LATISSIMUS DORSI

The "lats" as it is often referred to is a broad thin muscle that runs from the top of the hips and low back to the upper arm where it inserts beside the attachment of the pectoralis major. This is the muscle that sticks out underneath the armpit and gives body builders the V-shape in their trunk. You won't be able to feel the muscle on the back, but you'll be massaging it regardless. You can feel a part of this muscle on yourself by wrapping your hand around the back part of your armpit and squeezing the outer edge.

THE ROTATOR CUFF MUSCLES

There are four muscles that run from your shoulder blade to your humerus bone. They go all around the shoulder joint like a sleeve or cuff. The ligaments that hold the shoulder in place are very lax. As a result, these muscles have the job of keeping your humerus in the shoulder joint.

Supraspinatus. This rotator cuff muscle lies on the back of the scapula above the spine of the scapula. It is partly responsible for lifting the arm upwards (abducting the arm). It is somewhat difficult to palpate because it lies under the upper trapezius, but this cord-like muscle can be felt when firm pressure is used.

Infraspinatus. This rotator cuff muscle lies on the back of the scapula below the spine of the scapula. It makes your arm turn outward (external rotation). It is a flat muscle, but you can feel tight fibers within the muscle by firmly strumming across the fibers with your fingertips.

Teres Minor. This rotator cuff muscle lies on the back of the scapula below the infraspinatus and assists that muscle in performing external rotation of the arm. When palpating, it is difficult to distinguish it from the infraspinatus.

Subscapularis. This muscle lies on the underside of the scapula. It's not easy to access and massaging this muscle can be quite uncomfortable.

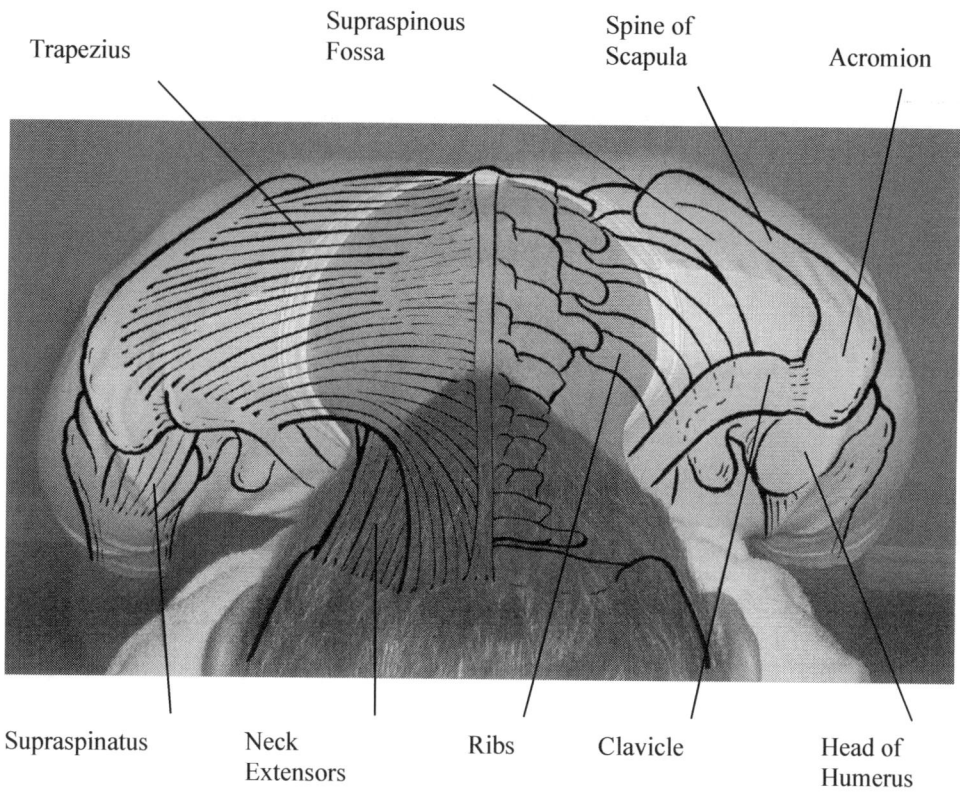

Trapezius   Supraspinous Fossa   Spine of Scapula   Acromion

Supraspinatus   Neck Extensors   Ribs   Clavicle   Head of Humerus

Arm muscles

DELTOIDS

The deltoid muscle, the "delts", is a large muscle that sits at the top of your arm. It runs from the collarbone and spine of the scapula down to a point about one third of the way down your humerus bone in an inverted triangle shape. The name is derived from Delta, a Greek letter that is shaped like a triangle. If you place the heel of your hand about a third of the way down your arm and wrap those fingers around your shoulder, your hand covers the deltoids and your fingers lie in the direction of the muscle fibers.

TRICEPS

The triceps (triceps brachii) is the big muscle on the back of the upper arm. It consists of three large sections of muscle, thus the name. It straightens the arm and therefore is involved in pushing movements.

BICEPS

This muscle (biceps brachii) lies on the front of the upper arm. Like the triceps it is divided into sections. It has two different attachments, thus the name. Whereas the triceps is involved in pushing actions, the biceps pulls objects by flexing the elbow.

FOREARM AND HAND MUSCLES

There are many muscles in the forearms and we will simply classify them into two groups. The forearm flexors and forearm extensors.

A band of fibrous tissue covers the tendons at the front of the wrist and holds them down. Below this fibrous covering is a space or tunnel that the tendons, nerves and blood vessels run through as they go into the hands. This is referred to as the carpal tunnel.

This is a very small space, so when the tendons get inflamed or when there is swelling in the wrist, the nerves may get compressed leading to pain, numbness and/or tingling in the hand and fingers. This is called *carpal tunnel syndrome*.

Symptoms usually start gradually, with frequent burning, tingling, or itching numbness in the palm of the hand and the fingers, especially the thumb and the index and middle fingers. Some carpal tunnel sufferers say their fingers feel useless and swollen, even though little or no swelling is apparent.

The symptoms often first appear in one or both hands during the night, since many people sleep with flexed wrists. A person with carpal tunnel syndrome may wake up feeling the need to "shake out" the hand or wrist.

As symptoms worsen, people might feel tingling during the day. Decreased grip strength may make it difficult to form a fist, grasp small objects, or perform other manual tasks. In chronic and/or untreated cases, the muscles at the base of the thumb may waste away. Some people are unable to tell between hot and cold by touch.

Fortunately, the majority recovers completely and only about 1% of cases result in any kind of permanent disability.

FOREARM FLEXORS

The forearm flexors flex both the wrist and the fingers. All the tendons of the flexor muscles come together and attach to a prominent bump on the inside of the elbow called *the medial epicondyle*. When this tendon becomes inflamed the condition is called *medial epicondylitis* or simply *golfer's elbow*. These muscles are involved in grasping motions. The muscle ends about two thirds of the way down the forearm and long tendons continue down the arm and attach into the hand and fingers. When you squeeze this muscle, especially the lower half, you should see the fingers curl.

FOREARM EXTENSORS

Whereas the flexors attach to the inside of the arm, the forearm extensor tendon attaches on the *lateral epicondyle* on the outside of the elbow. Tendinitis here is known as *tennis elbow*. The extensor muscles as a group are much smaller than the flexors and they run only about one third of the way down the arm before attaching into long thin tendons that insert on the back of the fingers.

SMALL MUSCLES OF THE HAND

There are numerous small muscles in the hand that are responsible for a variety of movements. The biggest group of these lie at the base of the thumb in an area called the *thenar eminence*. The other large muscle mass in the hand lies along the inside edge of the hand and is called the *hypothenar eminence*. There are a number of small muscles that run between the metacarpal bones that control finger movement. If you look at the palm of your hand, you'll be able to see how these bulge slightly below the web space of each finger.

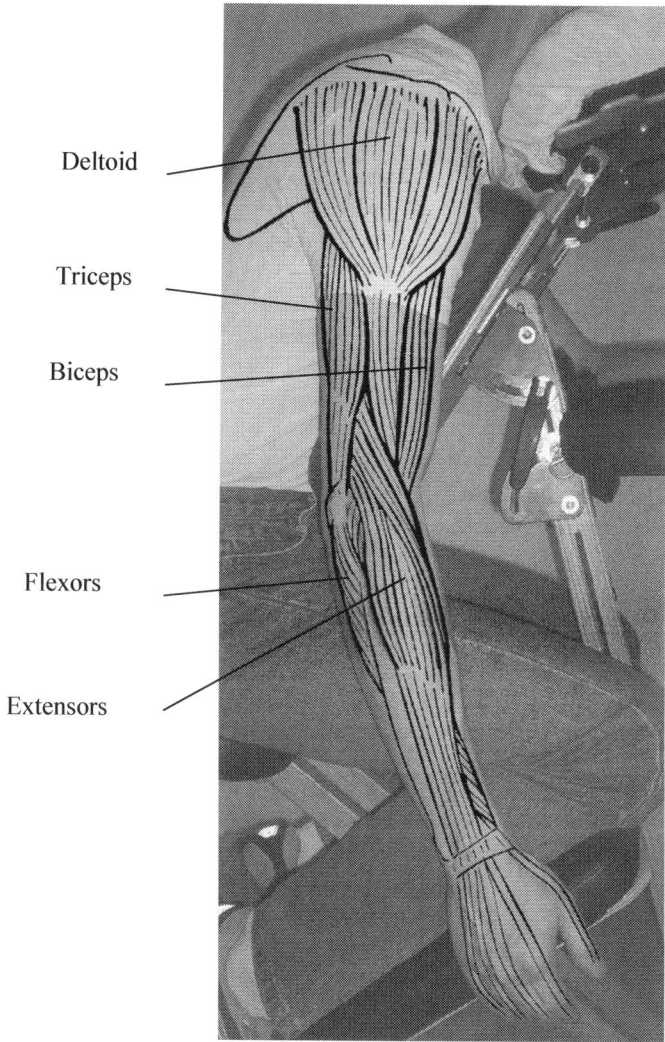

Deltoid

Triceps

Biceps

Flexors

Extensors

Lower body muscles

GLUTEALS

The gluteal area is usually referred to as the "bum" or "butt". These are strong powerful muscles around the hips. There are three gluteal muscles:

Gluteus maximus as the name implies is the largest of the three. It attaches to the sacrum and the back portion of the pelvis and wraps forward to attach into a long tendon-like structure called the *iliotibial band* (IT band) on the side of the thigh. This is the muscle that gives your backside a round curvy shape.

Gluteus medius is a fan-shaped muscle on the outside of the hip. It stabilizes the hip when you walk or when you stand on one leg. Underneath this muscle is the *gluteus minimus*. This muscle looks and acts like a mini-version of the gluteus medius.

HAMSTRINGS

The hamstring muscles (there are three of them) sit on the back of the thigh. At the distal end they attach on each side of the leg below the knee. The other end inserts into your "sitting bones". If you sit on a hard chair and rock your pelvis around a little you'll notice yourself rolling over two bony bumps that support your weight. These are your sitting bones or *ischial tuberosities* as they are called by anatomists.

QUADRICEPS

On the front of the thigh is the quadriceps. As the name implies, there are four muscles in this group. These are large, strong muscles that essentially wrap themselves around the thigh bone (femur). They work to straighten the knee, so they are involved in movements where your body changes levels, for example, standing from a sitting position or going up stairs. They also allow you to perform kicking movements.

CALF MUSCLES

There are two large muscles that make up your calf: The *gastrocnemius* (also referred to simply as the *gastroc*) and the *soleus*. The gastroc gives your lower leg that shapely look. It is located on the upper half of the lower leg. Underneath the gastroc and running further down the leg is the soleus. Both these muscles attach into the thick Achilles' tendon on the back of the ankle.

These muscles point your foot (plantar flexion). They allow you to raise up onto the balls of your feet and help push your body forward when you walk.

OTHER LEG MUSCLES

In the lower leg, there are three additional groups of muscles. They are described as being in compartments. There is an anterior, posterior and lateral compartment. These muscles work on the ankle, foot and toes.

The anterior compartment is in the lower leg just lateral to (or to the outside of) the shin bone. Place your hand flat over that part of your leg and pull your toes up toward your shin and you'll feel them contracting under your hand. When the attachments of these muscles become irritated and inflamed because of overuse, we call the condition *shin splints*.

Put your fingers on the very outside of the lower leg and press firmly as you move your fingers back and forth. You'll feel yourself strumming over the muscles of the lateral compartment (peroneals). These muscles help stabilize your ankle and prevent you from "rolling over" on your ankle and spraining it.

The muscles in the posterior compartment lie under the calf muscles and cannot easily be felt.

ILIOTIBIAL BAND

The one other structure in the thigh that we will be massaging is not a muscle. It is a very large, thick tendon called the *iliotibial band* or more commonly the *IT band*. This acts as a tendon for two muscles: the gluteus maximus that we've already discussed and another muscle on the front of the hip called the *tensor fascia lata* (TFL). This fibrous band runs down the lateral side of the thigh and inserts just below the knee.

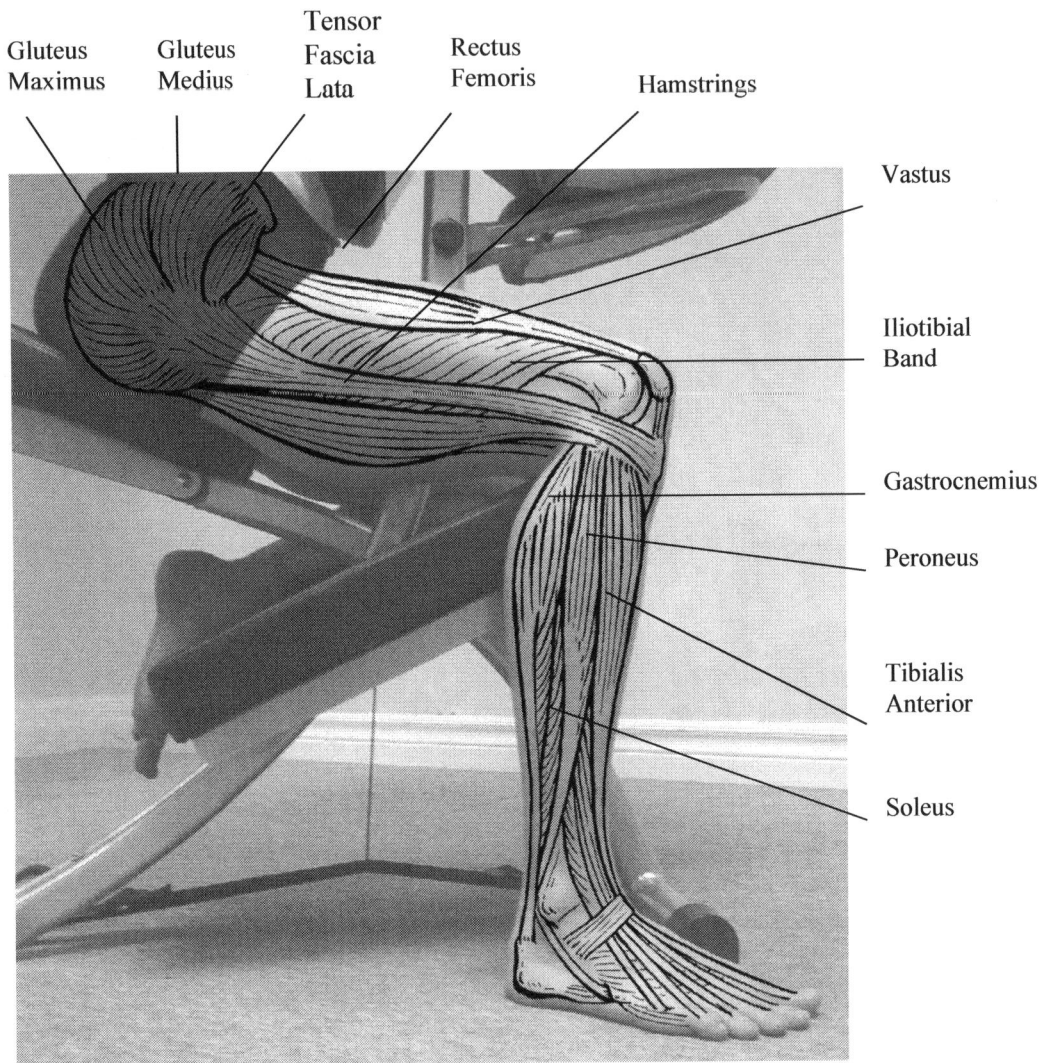

Gluteus Maximus

Gluteus Medius

Tensor Fascia Lata

Rectus Femoris

Hamstrings

Vastus

Iliotibial Band

Gastrocnemius

Peroneus

Tibialis Anterior

Soleus

Contraindications and Side Effects

Chair massage is extremely safe. However, it's important to note that there are some pre-existing conditions that can be aggravated by massage. It's important to be aware of these and to be able to screen out the customers for whom the massage will be inappropriate. This chapter will look at these contraindications and provide a system for screening potential customers. We'll also take a look at some of the potentially negative side effects that may result from your massage.

A search of medical and legal databases has turned up little evidence of harm arising from massage, especially in a normal healthy population. However, certain conditions may be present and could be aggravated or worsened by massage. In these situations massage is contraindicated. In other words, it would be inadvisable to massage customers with these conditions since the massage could possibly cause harm, aggravate, or worsen their condition.

When not to give a massage: Contraindications and precautions

Let's look at some of these contraindicated conditions. In short, all of the contraindications will generally fall into one of three categories:

1. Conditions where there is a risk of spreading infection

2. Conditions where the tissues are compromised or fragile

3. Conditions where we are unsure of the implications of doing massage

Before we get into detail however, here's a quick summary:

- Do not massage anyone who has a contagious infection, for example, the flu. Doing massage may exacerbate their symptoms and put you at risk of getting the infection and passing it on to others.

- Do not massage over inflamed joints or muscles. Signs of inflammation include redness, heat, swelling, pain, and a loss of movement. Massage will aggravate the inflammation.

- Do not massage a recent injury.

- Do not massage over open wounds or sores.

- Do not massage someone who is experiencing severe pain. Severe pain is an indication that there is some damage or inflammation in the body. If the person is experiencing severe pain they should be instructed to see their doctor or other health care professional.

Many times people with the above conditions think that massage will make them feel better when in fact the opposite is true. For example, when someone gets the flu they feel stiff and achy. Massage seems like something that will make their bodies feel better. But what will happen is that the flu symptoms will quickly get worse. The same thing applies for someone with an injury. People think that massage will make the pain go away when the massage will likely aggravate the inflammation and make the pain worse.

Notice in the list above that some contraindications would completely preclude the use of massage, for example, someone with the flu. This is what I might term a *general contraindication*. On the other hand, where the problem is confined to a small area, like a cut on their hand, massage can be done as long as you avoid the affected area. This is what is commonly known as a *local contraindication*.

Later we'll look at a screening process we can use to determine whether massage may or not be appropriate for any particular individual. For the time being, refer to this list. Before you massage anyone ask them if they have any of these conditions.

Contagious or infectious diseases

…in particular, any debilitating, systemic infections, whether they are bacterial or viral. For example, a cold or flu is a viral infection that is systemic, that is, it involves your whole body.

The concern here is three-fold:

1. The infectious agent weakens the customer's body. Any activity, including massage, puts further stress on the body, so the customer may feel the symptoms worsen. It is important that they rest.

2. The practitioners put themselves at risk by being exposed to the "germs".

3. There is a possibility of spreading the infection to other customers.

It is important to recognize that not all contagious infections are debilitating. In the case where it has no impact on their daily activities and they feel healthy, massage would be fine. For example, someone may have the HIV virus and be healthy and function normally. So this would not be a contraindication.

As well, not all infectious diseases are spread by touch or air. Many, like HIV, require the exchange of body fluids. If you use proper hygiene, which we'll talk about shortly, there is no danger of transmission. So as long as the person is healthy, there is little danger in doing the massage.

Always, if you have limited training and are not fully aware of the implications of doing massage on an individual, the rule is this:

If in doubt, don't.

Fever

Fever simply indicates that the person has a significant infection of some sort. For the reasons outlined above, it is best not to do massage until the person is healthy again.

Recent injuries

You do not want to massage recent injuries or areas that are healing because you will tear the fragile healing tissues, aggravate the injury and delay the healing process.

After you injure yourself, your body reacts by causing the area to become inflamed. As part of the inflammatory process, cells called *fibroblasts* move into the injured area and start laying down fibrous tissue to heal the injury. This fibrous tissue reconnects the edges of the wound. During the early stages of inflammation this fibrous bridge is very weak. Any additional stress to the site will cause the wound to separate and the pain and inflammation will get worse. In the long-term, this will also cause excessive scar tissue or scarring in the area.

What is a recent injury?

The textbooks say that the acute inflammatory phase lasts for 24 to 48 hours. But this time frame is based on physiological responses and doesn't have much relevance from a clinical perspective. As a general guideline, it would be best to wait a week before massaging an injured area. Of course, this would also depend on the extent or the severity of the injury. For example, someone who has a light strain of their calf muscle from playing baseball on the weekend is not going to be as much of a concern as someone who has been in a severe car accident.

As a general rule, most injuries will completely heal within six to eight weeks.

Recent surgeries

Treat a recent surgery the same way as you would a recent injury. The tissue has been surgically damaged and needs time to heal.

In the case of surgery, you may also need to consider the underlying condition, that is, the reason for the surgical procedure as well as the individual's current health status.

Acute inflammation

Avoid massaging over any areas where there are signs of acute inflammation.

Inflammation is a biochemical response that is involved in wound healing and reparative processes. All kinds of injuries respond by initiating an inflammatory response, so when you see inflammation, you can pretty much assume that the tissues have been damaged in some way. You don't want to massage the area for the reasons mentioned above in the *Recent Injuries* section.

The five typical signs of acute inflammation include:

1. Redness

2. Heat

3. Swelling

4. Pain

5. Loss of movement

Avoid areas where these signs are present.

Many people who are unaware of what inflammation is, actually use the term to refer to pain they may be experiencing. So when someone says, "My muscles feel inflamed," find out if any of those five signs are present to determine whether the area truly is inflamed.

Severe pain with or without movement

Pain is often associated with a recent injury and inflammation. Pain is a sign that the body's tissues are damaged in some way. Typically, if a person has pain with movement, this indicates that the problem is musculoskeletal. Pain without movement either indicates a severe musculoskeletal problem or is a sign of some other serious problem.

In any case, they should see a health professional to have the problem properly dealt with.

What is severe pain? Pain is very subjective. For our purposes we will consider pain severe if it limits activity or if it manifests itself on the person's face. For example, if someone lifts their arm up to the side and flinches or pulls their arm down to avoid the pain, or if someone can move their arm through a normal range of motion, but has a pained expression on their face as they do so.

Skin problems

These could include wounds, burns, bruises, rashes or other lesions. Some of these are obvious injuries to the skin, like cuts.

Wounds, burns (including sunburns), and bruises should be treated like an injury. We wouldn't want to do massage for the same reason that we would not massage any recent injury: We need to wait for the tissue to heal.

We want to avoid any skin lesions that are open or leaking fluids. Not only is the tissue likely fragile, but there is a risk of infection for both the customer and yourself. If anyone has a lesion that is bleeding, leaking, oozing, dripping, or weeping, the area should be cleaned up and the lesions properly covered with dressings.

There are all kinds of rashes that you may see on someone's skin. Rashes may or may not be infectious. For example, there is a range of skin conditions that we would refer to as *eczema*. These are non-infectious and are relatively benign. As long as their skin is not cracked or bleeding, it would be fine to massage these areas. However, some rashes may be contagious. For example, fungal infections are surprisingly common and can be contracted through skin contact.

Most customers are knowledgeable about any skin condition they may have, so don't be afraid to ask. They'll likely be able to advise you on whether it is harmless or not. Of course, our principal rule always applies: If you are in doubt, don't massage the customer. It's always in their best interest and yours as well.

Avoid any undiagnosed lumps. It could be something benign like some scar tissue or a fatty tumor (lipoma) in which case massage would be fine. On the other hand it could be something more serious like an area of infection that may be spread by the massage, or a cancerous tumor that may be fragile. Again, if you're unsure whether to massage the area, don't.

Unable to sit comfortably in the chair

If the person can't sit in the chair comfortably for any reason, don't massage them. Firstly, if they are not comfortable they are not going to be able to relax. Secondly, if it is pain that is preventing them from sitting comfortably, the problem is significant enough that they should be diagnosed and treated by a medical professional.

Other medical conditions...

I'm often asked questions about various conditions. These situations all involve people with various kinds of pathologies. I'll just touch briefly on some of the most common issues that students inquire about.

Important note: I want to reiterate that doing massage for an average healthy person carries very little risk. The risk of harm or complications rises when working with people who suffer from various medical conditions.

Once you begin working with populations that have more serious health problems, there are numerous factors that enter into the decision to massage these individuals. My personal feeling is that these populations present problems that are beyond the scope of practice of chair massage. If you decide to massage people with various kinds of pathologies, then you should be adequately trained and be familiar with the conditions you are dealing with as well as the implications or repercussions of doing massage for people with these conditions:

THROMBOPHLEBITIS OR DEEP-VEIN THROMBOSIS

If anyone has blood clots or a clotting disorder, like thrombophlebitis or deep-vein thrombosis, avoid massage of the legs. Furthermore, have the customer put their feet flat on the floor rather than on the shin rests.

This kind of situation is relatively rare, but is quite dangerous. I'll go into a little detail here simply because one of the few reported cases of harm through massage is the result of a clot being dislodged in the leg.

Clots are most likely to occur in the legs. A person is at risk if there is any inflammatory disorder of the blood vessels. However, it most commonly occurs when blood pools in the veins, which triggers blood-clotting mechanisms. For example, the pooling may occur after prolonged bed rest following surgery, or after a debilitating illness, such as heart attack, stroke, or fracture. If someone has any of the following conditions, they are at higher risk:

- Over the age of 60

- Recent accident, surgery, or other trauma

- Coronary artery disease

- Smoking

- Pregnancy

- Obesity

- Use of oral contraceptives

- Family history of clotting problems

Symptoms may vary widely. A mild case may have no symptoms. When symptoms do occur, they could include the following:

- Tenderness and redness in the affected area

- Pain and swelling in areas drained by the vein where the blood clot is located

- Fever

- Cramps

- Rapid heart beat

- Sudden, unexplained cough

- Joint pain and soreness

The problem with clots is that massage can actually dislodge them from the walls of the veins and send them into circulation. The clot travels through the circulatory system until it hits a narrow blood vessel. This usually occurs in the lungs. The lung's blood supply gets blocked, causing the affected part of the lung tissue to die. This could be potentially fatal.

VARICOSE VEINS

Varicose veins are the large, distended and twisted veins that you occasionally see in people's legs. They seldom occur in the upper body. Most varicosities occur in the superficial veins and for many people are simply a cosmetic problem. If your client does not have pain or discomfort in their legs, then it is probably fine to massage over the varicosities.

However, if the customer has symptoms of pain or discomfort in their legs, then it is likely best that you don't massage the legs. These symptoms may range from a feeling of tiredness or heaviness of the legs to more severe problems like ulcers in the legs or feet.

MULTIPLE SCLEROSIS

Typically there are no significant concerns in mild or moderate cases of multiple sclerosis (MS). Occasionally customers may report extreme fatigue following massage and may need time after the massage to sit and rest before continuing their activities.

IMPLANTS FOR IV MEDICATION

For people who need regular IV medication, catheters are implanted to facilitate delivery of the medication. There are two common types of implants that you may come across. One is installed in the arm. These are often referred to as PICC lines. There is a tube that runs up through the arm veins toward the heart. In this case, you want to avoid contact with the implant by avoiding massage to the arm and that side of the neck.

Another common type of line is implanted in the chest. These catheters are usually known by their brand names such as a Hickman line or Groshong catheter. Because these are installed on the chest, the person may not be comfortable putting their weight on the extruding plastic parts. You may need to get the person to sit upright or support the area around the device with a rolled towel to take weight off the implant itself.

STROKE PATIENTS

As long as the patient is stable, massage should be fine. There are often mobility issues however, and getting in and out of the massage chair may not be feasible. In addition, communication may be difficult where there is some cognitive impairment.

HEART ATTACKS

Like stroke patients, as long as their condition is stable, massage should not pose any significant risk. Strong compression to the trunk can cause pressure changes within the thorax that can alter blood pressure and cardiac output. For this reason, you may want to take a more gentle approach to compressions to the back.

CANCER PATIENTS

It is difficult to speak in generalities when it comes to cancer. There are numerous kinds of cancer with various presentations. Although generally speaking, massage will not increase the spread of cancer, there are many considerations including the health status of the patient, fragility of tissues, especially at tumor sites, and the interaction of massage with the treatments they may be receiving, such as radiation therapy.

For a detailed reference, see *Massage Therapy & Cancer* by Debra Curties.

There is often a concern that someone taking pain medication can't feel your massage and will be unable to tell you if you are massaging too deeply. This fear is largely unfounded. Pain relievers reduce pain sensation; they do not typically interfere with touch and pressure sensation.

More significant than the issue of the customer being able to give feedback about pressure is the reason for taking the medication in the first place. That is, do they have a recent injury or severe pain that would contraindicate your massage? Another lesser consideration is that many pain relievers have an anti-clotting agent – many are taken purposely as "blood thinners." As a result, people taking pain medication regularly or in larger doses may be more prone to bruising. Use moderate pressure for their first massage. Then monitor their response to the massage and adjust your technique appropriately.

The screening process

For a healthy individual, massage is extremely safe. When the massage is performed properly and you elicit feedback from the customer there are seldom any negative side effects. The side effects that may occur are infrequent and minor. We'll discuss some of the most common ones shortly.

We've looked at a variety of conditions that are contraindicated for massage. These conditions can be aggravated by massage or there is some increased risk of harm that may arise to the customer or even you as a practitioner.

It's important to identify people with contraindications so that we can either modify our massage or put off doing the massage altogether.

To do this, we use a systematic screening process with every client. We do this screening to determine whether or not massage is appropriate for each individual.

It would be impossible to screen for every conceivable condition that may have an impact on our massage. However, the screening process we've come up with weeds out most people in a healthy population for whom the massage may pose some risk.

The screening process is very simple to use, but it must be done consistently in the same way for each customer. You do not need to have a background in pathology to determine whether the massage will be safe or not.

There is one rule that you must keep foremost in your mind through the screening process and that is:

"If in doubt, don't."

OR

"If in doubt, refer out."

You can't hurt someone or aggravate their condition by not massaging them. So if you are ever in doubt, tell the person that given what they've told you, it is best that they see someone with appropriate training. You want to make sure that they get the best possible care. This is for their personal safety and wellbeing.

Not all situations are black and white. Oftentimes, there will be gray areas. Always use good common sense and always err on the side of caution.

The screening process is outlined in figure xx. Use the suggested wording or rewrite it in a way that feels comfortable for you. Practice going through this process and role-play with friends so you can see how it applies to a wide range of situations.

Keep in mind that this process I'm describing is simply a screening. It is designed only to qualify whether or not it is appropriate and safe for the person to get a massage. I'm not trying to get a comprehensive health history with this procedure. I'm simply filtering.

Note: If you have the time to take a comprehensive health history, then by all means feel free to do it. A thorough intake interview would also be necessary if you are doing treatment-specific work and your training allows you to utilize the knowledge you obtain for treatment planning.

Be sure to do the screening before setting your customer up in the chair. You don't want to spend the time required to get them comfortable in the chair if you can't proceed with the massage. More importantly, you don't want to create the expectation that they will get a massage when in fact the massage is contraindicated. Their reaction is likely to be: "Don't tell me we can't do it. You've got me all comfortable in this chair. You might as well go ahead with the massage now that I'm here." Now you're in a situation where you've got to extricate them from the chair.

It's much better to do the screening before they've invested time in the process. Introduce yourself and immediately go into the screening. Start off like this:

"Hi. I'm so glad to meet you. My name is Eric. And your name is? Okay. Before we start I need to ask you a few questions. I just need to find out if you have any health conditions that might interfere with me being able to give you a massage today."

As you do your brief introduction, look at the customer for visual signs that might indicate that massage shouldn't be done. For example, are they limping? Does their movement appear to be restricted in any way? Do they have a pained expression on their face? Do they look relatively healthy? Do they look flushed or feverish? Are they showing any signs of cold or flu?

Look for any visual signs that might indicate that they are less than healthy.

Then you can proceed with the screening. Let me go through the features of the process with an explanation of why we do it in this particular way..

We'll start by asking them three initial screening questions. Ask these first questions one at a time and wait for them to respond before moving onto the next. The three initial questions are:

1. Have you had any recent injuries?

2. Are you experiencing any severe pain?

3. Do you have any skin conditions that I should be aware of, such as…(give your customer several examples)

We want to know if they have any recent injuries to determine if there are any areas of tissue damage or acute inflammation. Notice that I've qualified the question of injuries with the word *recent*. Because I'm not doing a treatment-specific massage, I don't really need to know about their entire health history. I just need to determine whether they have any contraindications. If you ask the question in an open-ended way, be prepared to spend the time hearing the entire history of their body. People love to talk about their "war wounds." If they are not sure what recent means, then give them a time frame. Say, "…within the past week."

Severe pain indicates tissue damage, inflammation or possibly a more serious disorder. Again, for the purposes of screening, I do not need to know about every pain they have. I just need to know if the pain indicates a condition that I should avoid. So I specifically ask about *severe* pain.

Lastly, I want to know if they have any skin conditions that would be contraindicated. I usually preface this question by pointing out the areas of the body I'm going to massage. For example, I might say, "I'm going to be doing some massage to your arms, back, shoulders and neck today. Do you have any skin conditions in these areas…" As I mention the body parts I'm going to be massaging, I gesture to them with my hands. I do this to reinforce in their minds the areas I'm going to be massaging because they may be a little nervous or may be eager to get in the chair and are only half listening to my words.

I point out the areas I'm going to be massaging when asking this question to once again pinpoint contraindications. For example, I don't need to know that they have *Athlete's Foot*. I'm only concerned about skin conditions in the areas that I'm massaging.

I also give them examples of what I mean by skin conditions. Big pores or a coarse complexion is not something I need to know about. So I'll give specific examples of the information I'm looking for. I may say, "I'm going to be doing some massage to your arms, back, shoulders and neck today. Do you have any skin conditions in these areas, like bruises, cuts or rashes."

If I get a positive response to any of these three initial questions, then I need to explore the issue further. There are two additional pieces of information I'll need to know to determine whether or not I can proceed with the massage:

1. Is the injury, pain or lesion in an area I'm going to be massaging? If it's not, then I can likely proceed with the massage without incident. If it is, then I need to determine whether it is confined to an area that I can avoid without interfering with the massage.

    Get the person to physically pinpoint the area that is affected. For example, the back is a very large area. If they say they have pain in their back, it could be anywhere. Get them to point to the involved area or trace the edges of the problem with their finger so you know exactly where it is.

2. How severe is this particular problem? That is, is it severe enough to interfere with my ability to safely do massage for the person? This can be a gray area. What exactly is severe pain? It all seems quite relative. For example, someone may have sunburn. If there is just a little redness, then it may just be fine to massage, but if it's quite red then it should probably be avoided.

    As a general rule, if it interferes with their daily activities or movement or if it creates a pained expression on their face, then it can probably be considered severe. So if they complain of severe pain in their shoulder, get them to move the arm through a full range of motion. If they can't move it comfortably through a normal range or if they grimace as they go through the range, then it's probably best to avoid that area.

Be sure to get through each question individually. Oftentimes, I see practitioners explore a recent injury that the customer mentions, only to forget to ask about severe pain or skin lesions.

Don't be afraid to refuse to do the massage if you feel it is inappropriate. You are doing this in their best interests, so there is no reason to feel bad. It would be a good idea to role-play this situation with a friend so that you feel comfortable refusing to do a massage when the situation arises. Many people mistakenly think that rubbing their sore or painful areas will make them feel better, but we know that's not necessarily the case.

Just because you are refusing to do the massage this time doesn't mean they can't have a massage in the future. Make this clear to them. I'd say something like:

"It seems that you have some condition today that is beyond my scope of practice. I would suggest seeing a qualified health professional to get that assessed and properly treated. When you're feeling better, I'd be happy to see you back here for some massage."

If they pass the screening and you feel that it is appropriate that they receive massage then proceed with your session. Refer to the next chapter for more information on getting them prepared for the massage.

Side effects

Although seated massage is extremely safe, there are some possible negative side effects. They seldom happen and they are certainly not life threatening.

Stiffness

One of the most common side effects of the massage is stiffness the day following the massage. The massage techniques are designed to put a little bit of a stretch on the muscle. The massage stretches the muscles in ways that they don't normally stretch. Because of this, a customer may feel like they've worked out a little and may have a little stiffness that is similar to post-exercise soreness. Typically, they won't feel this immediately after the massage, but instead, they will feel the stiffness when they get out of bed the next day.

This stiffness will be more likely to occur when the customer:

- Feels tenderness during the massage

- Is relatively sedentary

- Has not had massage before or gets massage infrequently

It is unlikely to occur when the customer:

- Does not experience tenderness with the massage

- Exercises regularly

- Gets regular massage

📄 Side note...Delayed Onset Muscle Soreness

The stiffness and tenderness that someone feels the day after a massage is referred to as delayed onset muscle soreness (DOMS). People who have just started exercising are familiar with the sensation. They feel great right after they've exercised, but wake up the next day stiff and tender. The soreness is generally at its worst within the first 2 days following the activity and subsides over the next few days.

DOMS is a result of microscopic tearing of the muscle fibers. It takes time, hours or even days, for the low-grade inflammation to fully develop. You can liken this process to getting sunburn. You don't realize you've been in the sun too long until the inflammation starts to peak hours later and you start to see the redness in your skin.

This is much different than the acute pain of a pulled or strained muscle. A muscle tear is usually felt as a sudden, sharp pain that occurs during activity. The typical signs of acute inflammation often accompany these kinds of injuries.

With exercise-induced DOMS, the symptoms usually disappear within three to seven days. Because massage puts much less stress on the muscle than exercise, massage-related DOMS usually doesn't last for more than 24 to 48 hours.

Common ways of treating the symptoms include pain relievers, hot baths, ice, vitamins (particularly C and E) and light exercise or stretching. However, none of these methods have been proven to help significantly. Like sunburn, it just takes time for the body to recover.

On a positive note, once your muscles adapt to the stresses of massage, usually after one or two sessions, DOMS is not likely to recur.

Fainting

Fainting is a phenomenon that seems to be unique to chair massage. When I first learned about chair massage I was told that one in 1,000 people would faint when getting a seated massage.

I did thousands of massages between 1993 and 1997. I kept waiting, with a certain level of anxiety, for someone to pass out. It never happened to me or anyone I had trained personally.

Then in 1998 when I started a professional training program in massage we experienced a series of fainting episodes in customers – up to ten occurrences within the year. We were quite baffled. I had been told that this fainting would happen when working particular points in the hand or if the customer hadn't eaten. But that was never the case.

So we began to interview anyone who had experienced a fainting episode to find commonalities that we could include in a screening process. Much to our dismay, there seemed to be very little in common between these people. Most were women. The ages ranged from 10 years to about 60. The fainting had occurred within a couple of minutes of starting in one case and in another at the end of a half hour massage. There was absolutely no association between these episodes and the part of the body we were massaging. The fainting did not seem to be related to low blood pressure or menstruation.

We put considerable time and energy into the problem. We knew a person faints when there is inadequate blood flow to their brain – when the blood pressure is not sufficient to pump blood to the brain.

We also knew that massage would decrease a person's blood pressure to a certain extent. There is no specific area or reflex zone that does this. It is simply a result of relaxation. When you are relaxed, your heart doesn't pump as vigorously as it normally does and your blood pressure drops. With table massage, even though the blood pressure decreases, it's not really an issue because the person is lying horizontally. The heart doesn't need to pump forcefully against gravity. With table massage, if the person feels lightheaded or faints, it will most likely happen when they sit or stand up after the massage is finished and before the heart has a chance to compensate for the lowered blood pressure.

With chair massage this occurs because the person remains upright and the heart must continue to pump blood against gravity toward the brain as the person relaxes. But the blood pressure regulation systems should be able to compensate or adjust for this.

If this was in fact the mechanism behind the fainting, we would expect this to be a gradual process and for the person to report feeling lightheaded or dizzy. And sometimes this did occur.

But these kinds of occurrences didn't seem that significant. We had lots of time to assist the person out of the chair and to position them on the floor or with their head between their knees until it passed.

What surprised us was that almost every fainting episode happened very quickly and with very little warning. A relaxation induced drop in blood pressure just couldn't account for this sudden and dramatic effect.

When we were discussing the issue one day, my senior trainer, Kam Toor, suggested that the fainting might be caused by the carotid sinus reflex. As we started to discuss this possibility, it made perfect sense.

This is a well-documented reflex that was first noted way back in 1866. It's sometimes referred to as the Weiss-Baker syndrome after the two researchers, Soma Weiss and James Porter Baker, who described it comprehensively in 1933.

There are baroreceptors (blood pressure sensors) in a blood vessel called the carotid artery that goes to the head. They help regulate the flow of blood to the brain. If they sense that there is a high level of pressure in the carotid artery then they initiate a reflex that quickly slows down the heart.

Symptoms usually occur with neck movement, such as while shaving or turning the head while reversing a car, or from wearing a too-tight collar. The result is severe lightheadedness and fainting.

It doesn't take a lot of pressure to the carotid artery to cause the reflex. And the heart slows down quickly and dramatically when the reflex is elicited. Doctors will test this reflex by applying a little pressure to the carotid sinus just below the angle of the jaw for just five seconds. Furthermore, some people seem to have a genetic hypersensitivity to this reflex.

Why is this fainting reflex triggered with chair massage?

When I first started teaching chair massage to larger groups of people, one of the most common mistakes I saw was the positioning of the face rest of the chair for the customer. Almost all students had a tendency to put the person's face too high on the face rest. Instead of supporting the forehead, the top of the pad came closer to eye level. And the sides of the face rest, instead of supporting the sides of the cheeks, came down to the sides of the neck.

So the face rest pad would be pushing into the carotid sinuses just below the jaw!

Once we recognized that, we became very strict about the adjustment of the face rest making sure the pad supported the face properly. In addition, before each massage, we had students ensure that there was clearance between the neck and the pad. Since that time, we have had almost no reported cases of fainting.

The first sign that a person is about to faint is dizziness or lightheadedness. Sometimes the customer may experience these symptoms and will not tell you. The most common indicator that they are not feeling well is squirming in the chair. If you see them moving around, stop and ask them specifically if they feel lightheaded or nauseous.

If a customer tells you that they are experiencing these symptoms as they are getting the massage it's best to get them out of the chair and have them lie on the ground. This helps ensure that there is sufficient blood flow to the brain. Being on the floor is also safe because if they pass out, they won't fall and hurt themselves.

Don't leave them in the chair to get a glass of water or a cold compress. Get them on the floor first.

Always ASSIST the customer out of the chair if they begin to experience symptoms. Stand behind the person and put one foot forward. Hook your elbows under their armpits and support some of their weight as they stand up. Stay behind them in this position and step away from the chair. Keep one leg in front of the other and support their weight as you lower them to the floor.

If they faint as you are getting them out of the chair, don't try to hold them up. They are dead weight. Let them slide down your body and fall with them. Most importantly, stop their head from hitting the floor.

If a customer faints as you are massaging them, keep them resting forward in the chair and support them with your hands so they don't fall off. Don't try to get them off the chair if they are unconscious.

No matter what the situation, **don't panic!** The fainting spell will pass. Stay calm. Gently shake the person and call their name. They will most likely regain consciousness within seconds.

The experience can be frightening if you've never seen it happen before. Their eyes will roll back into their head and they will gasp. They may start to convulse. Sometimes the convulsions are just a slight tremor or shake and sometimes it may appear as though the person is having a mild epileptic episode.

There are really no lasting effects from the fainting. They may feel a little queasy, but after a short time frame and once their blood pressure normalizes, they should feel fine.

Be sure to explain what has happened so that they understand that it was not something that happened as a result of the massage, but rather a simple reflex that was caused by some pressure to the front of their neck.

Lightheadedness and nausea

Although fainting is rare, especially if you're careful with the setup of the chair, lightheadedness and nausea are reported a little more frequently. This is a symptom of decreased blood flow to the brain. It could be caused by a low level activation of the carotid sinus reflex that we've discussed or could simply result from decreased blood pressure brought about by relaxation.

This is more likely to occur in circumstances that cause blood to be diverted from core circulation. In these situations, there is simply less blood for the heart to pump to the brain, so the effect is easier to elicit. Here are the situations you should be particularly aware of:

1. *If someone has just eaten a meal,* there will be a diversion of blood to the stomach and intestines to digest the food. There is less blood circulating to the muscles and other organs. That's why you will often feel tired after a big meal.

2. *If someone has just exercised without cooling down.* The blood in this case is diverted to the muscles. In exercise classes they typically have you do cool-down exercises at the end of your exercise session. In the cool-down exercises the instructor has you do light muscle contractions to force the blood out of the muscles and into circulation again. If someone sits in the chair without cooling down sufficiently, their blood pools in their muscles, especially in the legs, which are in a bent position. Don't massage anyone who has been exercising who is flushed, hot, actively perspiring, or breathing heavy. It is probably best to ask them to wait until they've taken a shower, which should give their blood flow ample time to normalize.

3. *If someone is very hot.* When you become heated, blood flow is diverted to your skin where the air can take the heat away from your body. Again, more blood in the skin means less blood in circulation to your brain.

The other situations where lightheadedness may be more likely to occur are if the person has low blood pressure or a history of fainting. You may want to include this as part of the screening process.

Nausea is another symptom of lowered blood pressure. In our experience, the nausea, like lightheadedness, does not go away if the massage continues. It is best to end the massage as soon as the customer reports either of these symptoms. Ask the customer to slowly get out of the chair. Assist them in doing so. Let them sit or lie down until the sensation subsides. Vomiting because of this nausea is extremely rare.

Headaches

Although headaches are sometimes relieved by relaxation massage, occasionally a customer will report that the massage causes a headache. This happens because of activation of **trigger points**. Trigger points are what people usually think of as knots in their muscles. They are areas where the muscle spasms in a very small area. Unlike a cramp where the whole muscle contracts, a trigger point only affects a few muscle cells and is only a few millimeters in length.

The interesting feature of these trigger points is that they can send pain traveling to different areas of the body, sometimes nowhere near the trigger point area itself. For example, there are trigger points in the trapezius muscle that can send pain into the base of your skull, your temples, or even your jaw. These trigger points can sit in your muscles for years without giving any indication that they are there. In this state, they are called *latent trigger points*. But physical or emotional stress can "trigger" the latent points and they become *active trigger points*. When active, they can refer pain, tenderness, and sometimes other unusual symptoms to different areas in your body.

Sometimes the massage can put stress on latent trigger points and activate them. The trigger point then starts referring pain, usually into the head, but sometimes into the shoulders and arms. This is not a permanent pain. You haven't injured the person. Once the trigger point "settles down" the pain will stop. This process could take minutes or hours. Putting heat over the neck muscles will usually help the trigger point relax more quickly.

It would be wise to suggest that the customer see a massage therapist or other healthcare professional who specializes in treating myofascial trigger points. Someone with the proper training can eliminate these trigger points in the muscle so that they do not cause recurring pain.

Preparing for the Massage

We're almost ready to start massaging. Before we set up the chair and begin, however, let's look at just a few issues around the massage and customer management.

Hygiene

As a practitioner, you need to practice proper hygiene to prevent the spread of any pathogens (disease causing organisms) including viruses, bacteria, fungi and protozoa. The concern is not just that you might "catch something," but also that you may pass pathogens onto your other customers.

Typically you are working through the clothing and there is little skin-to-skin contact. This alone minimizes the risk of spreading pathogens. Nevertheless, you need to take precautions.

The single best defense to spreading infectious organisms is simply hand washing. Be sure to wash your hands before and after each massage. Wash the fronts and the backs of the hands thoroughly. Also be sure to wash your hands after blowing your nose or after coughing or sneezing into your hands.

Since you will most likely be on-site and won't always have access to a sink, it is a good idea to carry an adequate supply of disposable hand wipes. The wipes should have some anti-microbial agent. Wipes with alcohol will serve this purpose.

There is a wide range of wipes available on the market. They have different disinfectant agents and have various degrees of wetness. Some of them smell pleasant and some smell distinctively chemical. Make sure you sample the wipes to find a product that meets your needs before buying large quantities.

We suggest wiping your hands in the presence of the customer. Getting germs is a concern of many people. Wiping your hands in front of them demonstrates in a tangible way that you are aware of the importance of proper hygiene.

As an alternative to wipes, you could use an anti-microbial liquid. These are effective, but the customer may or may not be aware that the stuff you are putting on your hands is a disinfecting agent and not just hand lotion. Your customer will likely feel more at ease if they see you physically wiping your hands with something.

Under normal circumstances, you should not come into contact with body fluids like blood, urine, feces, vomit, etc. If you should have any such spills on your chair it is important to disinfect your equipment. Wash your chair with soap and water and disinfect with a 10% bleach solution (one part bleach to nine parts water) or use a commercially available disinfectant solution. It is suggested that you use rubber or latex gloves.

If any body fluids come in contact with your skin wash immediately with soap and water and consider disinfecting the skin with a 10% bleach solution or commercial disinfectant. In the remote situation where body fluids come into contact with open wounds you may have, you should flush the wound with hydrogen peroxide or a 10% bleach solution.

Face rest covers

It is important that you clean the face rest for each client. You can simply use the same disinfectant wipes that you use for your hands. We haven't noticed any significant degradation of the vinyl as a result of doing this.

We don't suggest that the customer put their face directly on the vinyl. Most customers will feel uncomfortable about this even if it has been disinfected. We suggest using a face rest cover that is changed with each customer.

You can cover the face rest with either cloth covers (flannel and cotton ones are available commercially) or disposable ones.

The cloth covers are usually fitted for the face rest. Some are elasticized and others just drape over the face rest. Make sure that the cover is large enough to cover your face rest, especially with shrinkage after washing. We have seen some cloth covers shrink significantly. As a result, they end up fitting very poorly and unfortunately restrict the size of the hole in the face rest.

The cloth covers should be changed for every customer. To disinfect them, wash them in hot water with bleach.

The cloth covers provide good protection for the vinyl on your chair by acting as a barrier for oils from the customer's face. They are soft and feel comfortable against the skin. A small drawback is simply that you may need to stock and carry large numbers of these with you when working on site. For this reason, many practitioners prefer to use disposable face rest covers.

There are a number of options for disposable covers:

You can purchase covers that are specifically designed to be used with the face rests. They simply look like a square of soft paper with a "T" cut into one side. These are available at most massage supply stores. These will be the most expensive of all the disposable covers.

From conversations with practitioners, most common type of cover used is simply paper toweling. Practitioners simply tear off two of the perforated sheets, split them part way down the middle and lay them over the face rest. I've seen other practitioners use Kleenex or even J-clothes as disposable covers.

One of the drawbacks of using these kinds of disposable covers is that they are flat and tend to shift around or slide off the face rest. This is especially problematic if you get the person to sit up during the massage. However, some of these covers may be large enough to tuck into the sides of the face rest to secure them in place. Another disadvantage is that they often obscure the hole in the face rest. This is not an issue for the customer, but makes it difficult for the practitioner to determine where exactly the customer's face should be positioned when setting up the face rest.

Many practitioners use 21" bouffant caps as disposable covers. These are the bonnets that are used in hospitals – essentially as hairnets. They fit the face rest well and are elasticized so they won't fall off. You'll need to cut a slit up the center so that the customer can breathe. These are available at most medical supply stores and commercial kitchen supply stores. When bought in quantity, they can cost as little as five to ten cents each, so they are very inexpensive as disposable covers.

The drawback is that they are porous, so that there is some contact with the vinyl. From the standpoint of infection control, the face rest is disinfected for each customer, so hygiene isn't an issue. However, many people will find that their faces start to feel itchy if they are lying in the face rest for extended periods of time.

So what are my personal suggestions in terms of face rest covers? My preference is the cloth covers, especially the flannel ones, because they are comfortable for the customer and they cover the vinyl well. However, the disposable covers are more convenient. I have a preference for the bouffant caps, but each kind of disposable cover has its pro's and con's, so I wouldn't say they are necessarily the best option.

What to wear

You need to wear loose comfortable clothing in which you can easily move. Very tight pants, short skirts or high heels just don't work very well. Wear a short sleeve shirt because many of the techniques you'll be learning will involve the forearms and elbows. Having the arms bared will help improve your sensitivity.

Although small jewelry is fine to wear, big bulky rings and necklaces can get in the way. It's probably best to leave your jewelry at home. Rings can usually stay on the fingers. Because you'll be using the fists for a number of techniques, if your rings have stones, turn the ring around so that the stone is on the palm side of the hand.

Because of the nature of some of the techniques, you'll want to have your heel secured in a shoe. Most sandals do not secure the foot sufficiently and as a result won't allow you to use your body effectively.

Dress appropriately for the type of customer you serve. You are going to dress very differently working at a Rave (all night dance party) than you would if doing massage at corporate headquarters. People will judge you by your looks, so be sure to present yourself in a way that is a true reflection of your professionalism.

Err on the side of caution and dress conservatively. At the risk of sounding prudish, I'd say: no jeans, halter-tops, bare midriffs, low cut tops, short shorts or mini skirts. I've personally had a massage where the therapist took his shirt off because he was too hot. Please don't do that.

It's also best to avoid using perfumes or colognes. Some people have sensitivities to these things. Furthermore, some corporations even have policies that forbid perfumed products on the premises.

Cut your nails

Unfortunately, you can't do massage with long nails. You'll find yourself modifying your technique to avoid sticking them into your customer's body. This will put unnecessary stress to the joints of your fingers. It will also hinder you in using proper technique and as a result you won't be able to target the muscles properly.

I know some practitioners hate to part with their nails, but they have to be cut short – the shorter the better. If you hold your palms toward you, you should not see nails peeking up above the fleshy parts of your fingers.

Client Communication

Consent

Getting consent from your customer is vitally important. You want to do this to avoid misunderstandings and meet your customer's needs in the best way possible. If you are a regulated professional, it may even be required by law.

Getting consent is a very simple process. Simply give your customer a brief outline of what you propose to do during the massage. Then ask them if they are okay with the proposed massage or whether they would like you to do things differently.

For example, you might say:

"I'm going to do 15 minutes of massage to your back, neck and shoulders. I will spend most of that time focusing on your neck and shoulders since that's where you've mentioned you're feeling tight. If anything feels too painful or uncomfortable, please let me know right away. I want you to be able to relax completely. How does that sound? Is that okay with you or is there anything you'd like me to do differently?"

Some practitioners are even more direct in verbalizing consent. They may specifically ask:

"Do I have your consent to proceed with the treatment I've outlined?"

Personally, that's a little too formal for me. But it really doesn't matter how you phrase it. What is important however is that you actually get their verbal (or written) permission to go ahead with the massage you've described to them.

Then make sure you do exactly as you've outlined unless they want to change things once the massage is underway.

In going through this consent process, your customers know exactly what to expect. There are no surprises. For example, they won't be shocked that you are touching their bum when you are doing the "gluteal compressions."

It also ensures that your massage meets their needs. You may find, for example, that once they hear your plan, they may decide that they would like more focus on a particular area than you have indicated you'll do.

As well, it gives them an opportunity to express their concerns or reservations. If you planned on doing some scalp massage and they don't want their hair messed up, then they can tell you.

Lastly, it gives them a feeling of control over the situation, which will help them to relax.

Right of refusal

The client has the right to refuse the massage practitioner's services. They can refuse or stop the session anytime even if you received prior consent.

You, as a practitioner, also have the right to refuse to provide a service, but only if you have just and reasonable cause. You must be able to explain the reason for refusal to your customer. You are bound by human rights laws. You cannot discriminate against customers on the basis of culture, ethnicity, age, gender, belief, or sexual orientation. You can, however, restrict your business to specific age, gender groups, or to specific conditions as long as this is consistent and not applied arbitrarily.

Here are examples of some situations where you could refuse to provide massage:

- The customer has a condition that you feel is beyond your scope of practice.

- The customer has a condition that could be worsened by massage.

- The customer is sexualizing the relationship.

- You feel that your safety is in question.

Here are examples of some situations where you could not refuse to provide massage:

- The customer is gay.

- The customer is Jewish (or any ethic group).

- The customer is HIV positive.

If you are regulated under State or Provincial legislation, there may be specific guidelines around this issue that you would have to adhere to.

Confidentiality

In the course of your business, you customer may tell you information about their health or their personal lives. This information is private and it would be unethical to discuss this information with others. If you wish to discuss a customer's personal or health information with a friend or colleague, do not mention their name or discuss details that would reveal their identity.

Obtain written consent from the customer before sharing their information with third parties. It's your job to safeguard the confidentiality of all customer records. Their information should only be released at their request or if required by law or court order. Be sure to keep a written record of any situation that requires the release of their confidential information.

Name, address and telephone numbers are considered to be public information and the sharing of this kind of data is generally not covered under most privacy regulation unless, of course, it is associated with other personal or health information.

Again, licensing boards may have specific guidelines around the use and sharing of customer information that you need to follow.

Prior to the massage

This is the first time many people will have had massage. They are taking a risk in trying something new and are likely nervous about the experience. For this reason, it is important to do as much as possible to make them feel comfortable.

The most important thing you can do to help them relax is to be very clear as to what they can expect and what they are to do. You want to avoid any uncertainty or ambiguity.

Summarize what you are going to do in the massage so that there are no surprises. It's useful to point out the areas that you are going to be massaging on your own body so they can visually see where they are going to be touched.

Get consent. Find out if what you are planning to do is OK with them. All you have to say after describing your proposed massage is, "How does that sound to you? Is there anything you'd like to change or do differently?"

This puts them in control and ensures that they are going to have their needs met.

Always provide clear instructions on getting into and out of the chair. It may seem self-evident to you, but people manage to sit in the chair in some very unique ways.

Let them know that you welcome feedback during the massage and if they feel uncomfortable for any reason during the massage to let you know.

Always, do your screening before the customer gets into the chair. If you get your customer in the chair and make them comfortable, they are going to feel very disappointed if you tell them that you can't do the massage. So find out if the massage is appropriate for the individual before they sit down.

As a professional courtesy, offer to take their glasses and put them somewhere safe. If they are carrying a purse or parcels, put them directly under the chair so that the person can relax knowing that they are safe. Alternatively, place them in front of the chair, but out of your way, so they can see their stuff through the face rest hole. Let them know that you'll keep your eye on their valuables and won't let them out of your sight.

If you want them to remove clothing, like a heavy sweater or jacket, ask them if they would mind removing it. Don't demand it. They may not feel comfortable removing that particular piece of clothing. For example, a woman wearing a suit jacket may only have a light camisole underneath.

If anyone is wearing a button up shirt or tie, ask them to undo the first button and loosen their tie. You don't want them to feel choked during the massage.

A note on setting up your chair...

In busy environments, position your chair so that the face rest is away from traffic. It will be somewhat quieter for the customer and they won't see feet walking in front of them. Removing awareness of the crowds as much as possible helps makes them feel a little more sheltered. In addition, facing your chair away from the crowds like this will prevent women in skirts from feeling exposed.

During the massage

Always look for signs that pressure is too deep. Signs would include: twitching, breath holding, body stiffening, guarding or tightening up.

Get feedback regarding your pressure. Through the 15-minute routine that you'll learn in this book, you'll see that we build the feedback requests right into the routine as though it were one of the techniques.

When eliciting feedback, don't ask them, "Is the pressure OK?" Ninety percent of the time they will say yes to avoid appearing to criticize you. Instead, elicit feedback giving them choices. For example: "Could this pressure be lighter or deeper?" This is the least intimidating way of getting them to respond honestly to you. You've given them only two choices. If the pressure is comfortable then they have to make a deliberate effort to tell you.

In noisy environments when it is difficult to hear what your customer is saying, use hand signals for feedback. Ask them to give you a thumb up for more pressure, a thumb down for less pressure and an okay sign when the pressure is just right.

Because this is the first massage experience for many customers, they are not sure how the massage should feel. They may ask you questions like, "Should this hurt?" or "How deep should it be?" Give them specific criteria that would indicate that the pressure is too deep. You might respond in the following way: "You may feel a little discomfort, but the massage should not feel painful. If you feel that the pressure I'm using makes you tense up or hold your breath, it's too deep."

Stay focused on the massage and your customer's experience as much as possible. Avoid talking to co-workers or passersby, don't answer your cell phone, and don't interrupt the massage to check your watch every couple of minutes.

Any particular massage may not feel that special to you. It may be your 10th massage of the day, the 200th massage of the month or the 1,000th massage of the year. I understand why you may lose interest or focus after seeing a couple of dozen people in rapid succession. It's easy to get distracted.

But you always have to remember that this massage is special to the person in the chair. It matters to them that you are focused and giving them the attention they deserve. Always keep that idea at the top of your mind.

After the massage

Let them know when the massage is finished. Otherwise, they won't know. There's nothing more stressful at the end of a massage than to have the practitioner disappear or stop massaging without telling you. The customer doesn't know if you've stepped away momentarily, have gone to the bathroom, or whether you've suddenly gotten ill and passed out. They don't know if they should get out of the chair or stay still. They certainly don't want to appear foolish by doing the wrong thing. It's an anxiety-inducing situation. So please, don't be a vanishing practitioner. Tell your customer the massage is over and give them clear instructions on getting out of the chair.

You can say something like, "Okay John, you're massage is over now. I want you to sit up slowly. Take a few seconds to come back to reality before you get out of the chair."

To make sure that you are meeting their needs, we suggest asking for feedback after each session. Asking closed ended questions like, "Did you like that? Do you feel good?" doesn't really give you any useful information. In addition, you are not likely to get useful feedback if you position your questions in such a way that the customer feels that they are criticizing you. For example, if you ask, "Is there anything in particular you liked about the massage? Anything you didn't like?" You are likely to hear, "I liked it all. It was all good." That may be good for our ego, but it doesn't give us the information we need to improve their experience.

One effective way of eliciting their preferences is the following questions: "What technique should I be sure to include in your massage next time? If I don't have enough time, what techniques would you want me to leave out?" It's a very non-threatening way to get useful feedback that will help you adapt your massage to their preferences next time around.

Make a note of any feedback or suggestions and be sure to incorporate these into your next massage with that particular individual.

Of course, you want to ask them to book their next appointment before they leave, but that's an issue we'll look at in the *Chair Massage Business* book.

The Massage Chair

The massage chair is an integral part of chair massage. Let's take a look at the chair, go over some of the features that you will want to consider in buying a chair and learn how to set it up for maximum comfort.

Why you must buy a chair

A massage chair is absolutely, positively indispensable if you are going to do chair massage. Why? Let's do a little history lesson to find out.

Seated massage has been performed for hundreds, no, make that thousands of years. Most Eastern forms of massage incorporate techniques where the receiver sits upright while work is performed on the neck, shoulders, scalp and back.

In this century there have been a number of practitioners who have utilized seated massage in a variety of settings including the workplace. Yet all this seated massage went on relatively unnoticed. Most practitioners hadn't heard of it. The media didn't care. The average person on the street would have given you a confused look if you suggested that they have a seated massage.

So what happened? Somebody invented a massage chair and made what was an invisible service into a "real" tangible product. It gave a face to the service and an industry was born.

A real life example: We were in a company for the first time doing chair massage. The employer paid for it. Several employees somewhat reluctantly walked into the boardroom for their massage. They entered the room and saw the massage chairs set up. Their eyes widened. "Oh!" one said in surprise. "This is a serious massage." Another one of the employees said, "I didn't think this was going to be a *REAL* massage."

You see, chair massage without the chair is just not a "real" massage.

If you are going to do chair massage, you need a massage chair.

What chair is the best chair? There's no such thing as a perfect chair. It hasn't been invented and probably never will be. Why? Because there are two competing factors that go into designing a chair.

On one hand, the chair needs to be designed with a wide range of adjustments. You want your chair to fit every body shape and size that might sit in it – from basketball players to the vertically challenged. You also want a chair that can be adjusted for your body size and shape. For example, you don't want a chair that is so low that you feel that you have to do the massage on your knees.

On the other hand, the chair needs to have as few adjustments as possible so that it is easy to use. It must have the fewest number of adjustments to make so it can be set up in a few seconds instead of several minutes. You don't want to spend more time setting up the chair than you do on doing the massage.

In short, it has to be designed for both the comfort of the customer and for the convenience of the practitioner. The customer and the practitioner have conflicting needs, so there are tradeoffs. For example, to create a chair that is quick to set up, the designer creates fewer adjustable pieces, which means that you can't make fine adjustments to make the customer perfectly comfortable.

There are now dozens of chairs to choose from. I've bought and tested pretty much every one on the market. If a chair comes out that has any unique design features, I usually pick it up right away. There are probably no more than half a dozen unique designs. Most chairs are simply knockoffs of the originals with some small variations.

We'll give you some of our recommendations based on our extensive use of these chairs and feedback from other practitioners. Suffice it to say that you should buy the best chair you can afford.

Many manufacturers of the low-end or cheaper massage chairs argue that because the massages are short that the chair doesn't have to be all that comfortable. I'm afraid that I'd have to disagree. Even five minutes in an uncomfortable chair can seem like hours. And if the customer is uncomfortable in the chair, it doesn't matter how good your massage is. They won't enjoy the experience.

There are other considerations in buying a low-end chair. Generally speaking, you get what you pay for. A more expensive chair typically has a five-year warrantee. The cheaper ones often have only a one-year guarantee. This gives you a sense of the projected life of your chair and the number of problems you will likely see. In addition, the less you pay, the less support you can expect to receive if something goes wrong. Companies that operate on the basis of price are more likely to go out of business. They may not always be around to service your chair through its lifetime.

Perhaps a more important issue is product liability. Larger manufacturers are usually smart enough and have the resources to invest in product liability insurance. Let's suppose you are using the chair and it breaks and injures someone. It's really the manufacturer and NOT you who are legally responsible. If the person takes legal action, the manufacturer has product liability insurance that should cover the incident. If they don't have product liability (most one person companies won't) then the lawyers will come after you.

Beyond that however, why would you want to put a customer at risk in the first place by putting them in a chair that may be poorly constructed?

Don't put yourself or your customer at risk for the sake of saving a couple of hundred dollars. Please invest in a good quality chair produced by a manufacturer that has been around and will stand behind their product.

Getting the perfect chair

Now, what chair should you buy? Although the perfect chair doesn't exist, there are some that come relatively close.

There are dozens of different models of massage chairs and we've field-tested most of them.

The Winner: ErgoPro

This is our favorite of all the chairs we've tested. The ErgoPro chair is manufactured by StrongLite. It strikes one of the nicest balances between customer comfort and ease of use. It has a wide range of independent adjustments and fits people of all sizes and shapes. It sets up and folds away in seconds. Even though it only weighs 19 pounds, it can hold some really giant people – up to 800 pounds – so you can be sure it won't fall apart. It comes with wheels so that you can easily pull it behind you.

Other great features: An independent height adjustment for the practitioner, so that you can adjust the chair to the best height for you. This is the only chair on the market that has this type and range of height adjustment.

As well, it is the only chair that has removable shin rests which allows the person to put their feet flat on the floor without having to spread their legs. This is a great feature when you are doing work with people who have knee problems, like recent surgeries or osteoarthritis, and is very useful if you are doing massage for the legs and feet while the person sits in the chair.

We like the little attention to details. For example, the corners of the seat are cut away so that even if you don't tilt the seat enough, the seat won't cut into the back of your customer's thighs. It's something that you wouldn't necessarily think as important, but if you've ever lost sensation in your legs after getting a seated massage in a chair that was poorly designed or adjusted, you'll understand how important little details like this can be.

Given the benefits, the StrongLite chair is the absolute best value for your money.

The Runner Up: Portal Pro

As a runner up to the StrongLite chair, we choose the Portal Pro from Oakworks. It's a sturdy chair with a good track record. I've had two of these chairs for almost ten years and despite a lot of use, they are still in great shape. They are true workhorses.

The chairs are very comfortable, but they don't have the same type of independent adjustments as the StrongLite chair. For example, you can't change the angle on the chest support and you can't change the height for yourself without changing the entire alignment of the chair.

Although I can get the seat flat in my older models, I haven't been able to get the seat to go flat in some more recent models. This could be a problem when you want to turn the person around and use the chair like a standard chair with their back against the chest support. For example, if you are massaging seniors or women in long tight skirts who can't lift their legs to straddle the chair, it would be nice to be able to flatten the seat so they could sit down comfortably facing you. Like the StrongLite, it comes with wheels so you can pull it along instead of carrying it.

Other thoughts...

All these chairs that I've mentioned so far have a "double action" face support or at least the option for this feature. This allows not just for tilt, but also for a horizontal forward and backward movement. This is pretty essential, so be sure that your chair has this capability.

Many face rests have a tilt only function. This can be problematic if your client has large breasts, a big belly or is simply thick through their trunk. In these cases, the thickness of their body pulls them further away from the chest support. When they drop their heads forward, it is nowhere near the face rest. Unless the face rest has the ability to translate forward to meet them, they are not going to be comfortable. In chairs with a tilt only head support, you'll usually have to take off the chest cushion to get them closer to the headrest. It's a less than ideal solution.

There are many other chairs that I wouldn't suggest you use. Too many for me to review here.

The bottom line: Stick with a good quality chair with a good basic design from a respected manufacturer.

Besides your training, the chair is the only other significant investment you'll need to make to get up and going with your chair massage business. If you can possibly afford it, we recommend that you buy the ErgoPro or possibly the Oakworks chair. If you buy either of these, you're assured that you will have a comfortable, easy to use chair from a reputable manufacturer that will last you for years and years. Your money will be well spent and you'll never have regrets.

Chair set up

One reason for getting the best chair possible is that you want your customers to feel comfortable. It doesn't matter how good your massage is, if they are not comfortable, they won't be able to enjoy the experience. They'll be too focused on their squished face, scrunched neck or painful back.

That's not to say that all you need is a good chair to make them comfortable. Setting them up in the chair in the right way is absolutely crucial. I can't emphasize this enough.

You have to be exacting and systematic in getting your customers in the chair. Just changing the tilt on the face rest a mere 10 degrees, for example, can make all the difference between them peacefully falling asleep or leaving the chair with a stiff neck.

Also, setting up the chair improperly may increase the risk of fainting in the chair. We discussed this in the *Side Effects* section, but we'll revisit the issue briefly when we look at adjusting the face rest of the chair.

Anatomy of a chair

Let's look at the various features of a massage chair. We'll look at the StrongLite Ergo, partly because it has a wide range of adjustments and partly because I really like it.

Chair height

The StrongLite chair has legs that telescope out to provide about eight inches of additional height. This adjustment is strictly for the practitioner and doesn't affect the customer's position or comfort. You can raise some chairs, but it usually changes the orientation of the various parts of the chair, in particular the orientation of the seat to the chest plate. The height adjustment here is unique in that it is independent. The ability to increase the height of the chair is particularly important if you are a taller practitioner.

Seat

You can tilt the seat to various degrees. Ideally, the seat should be tilted slightly forward for a couple of reasons. First, the forward tilt makes the person slide forward into the chest plate for better support. Second, because the thighs angle downward, if the seat is kept in a horizontal alignment, the corners of the seat cut uncomfortably into the back of the thighs.

However, you want to be able to put the seat into a horizontal position as well. That way, if someone cannot sit forward in the chair (like a senior with mobility problems), they can turn around, face backwards and use the massage chair like a standard chair.

Chest plate

Some chairs have tilt and height adjustments on the chest plate and others are fixed. The StrongLite has both capabilities.

The chest plate or chest rest should be positioned at least 90-degrees or more to the seat. This allows the bottom of the chest rest to give lots of support to the abdomen and support the back.

If the chest rest is too vertical, the person's back will be largely unsupported and will feel uncomfortable. If your client is pregnant or has a large belly, you can place the chest rest in a more vertical position since the abdomen itself provides support.

If you can adjust the height of the chest rest, like the StrongLite or QuickLite, position it in the middle of the trunk. You don't want it so high that it hits the front of the throat and you don't want it so low that the upper body has no support.

On most chairs the pads are attached with Velcro, so you can get a certain amount of adjustment simply by removing the pad and placing it where you need it. Although the pad should be oriented vertically, you can detach it and position it so that it is shorter and wider if necessary.

Most manufacturers sell *sternum pads* as an optional accessory. These are triangular shaped chest pads. They are designed to support more body weight at the sternum at the crest of the triangle. This could be used for someone with tender breasts, for example. You can also place the sternum pad horizontally for a pregnant woman so that the lower ribs bear more weight. This gives room for the belly under the crest of the triangle and supports the breasts above.

Shin rests

Every chair has shin rests. If someone has a knee injury or limited mobility in their knee, they can always place the foot flat on the floor beside or in front of the shin rest.

The StrongLite is unique in that it has removable shin rests. This makes positioning the feet flat on the floor more comfortable and keeps the customer's legs out of the way as you move around the chair. The removable shin rests are great for working on the lower body with the person positioned in the chair. It allows for better access to the legs and lets you use your body in a more efficient way.

Arm rest

The arm rests may have a height adjustment and/or tilt adjustment. Most people will feel most comfortable with the arm rest in a horizontal position. Tilt the arm rest one way or the other and it feels like your arms are sliding off.

Some chairs also have a height adjustment for the arm rest. If so, adjust the height so that the elbows bear some weight. Letting the arms hang puts a little too much stress on the shoulder girdle and can become uncomfortable.

Face rest

Almost every chair has a height adjustment for the face rest or face cradle. It is much preferable to get a "double action" face rest, rather than one with a tilt function only. With the double action face rests, you can adjust the tilt and it's also possible to get a horizontal back and forth movement of the face cradle.

This double action can be a really important mechanism for getting someone comfortable in the chair. You'll find it particularly useful for people who are big in the torso: large breasted women, people with large bellies or people who are barrel-chested. These people have a lot of mass between their center and the chest rest. As a result their head is further away from the face cradle. When they drop their head forward, it often falls short of the face rest unless you can move the face rest horizontally toward them.

Setting them up... step-by-step

It's important to be very systematic in setting up your customer. Here's a step-by-step approach that you should take for every customer.

First put the chair in neutral. By neutral, I mean a position where:

- The height is appropriate for you

- The seat is tilted downward slightly

- The chest pad is at least 90-degrees to the seat

- The arm rest is horizontal

- The face rest is dropped slightly

Greet your customer and do your screening. And remember to always do your screening before putting them in the chair. You don't want to get them all excited about getting a massage, get them all comfy in the chair and then tell them that they can't have one.

Then show the customer how to get into the chair. Physically go through the motions as you describe what you want them to do. You'll do this because they are likely a little nervous and not listening closely. Seeing you do it cues them visually. This will be a first time massage for many, so you don't want them to look or feel stupid trying to get into the chair.

So I might say something like this as I show them how to sit in the chair: "Just straddle the chair like this. Sit on the seat and slide your bum forward. Put your shins up on these pads like this. And just let your body relax forward completely against this chest support. Put your arms up here on the arm rest and I'll adjust this piece for your face and neck."

Then get out of the chair and repeat the exact same instructions as they sit into the chair. Make sure that they are doing as instructed and stop them if they rush through it.

It's important that you don't put the face rest in a position that they can put their head in immediately. They see it as a target and that's the first thing they aim for. When they do that, it interferes with their getting proper support from the chair. So please be sure that the rest of their body is well supported and in good alignment before even getting them close to the face rest. Notice in the picture of the chair in neutral position that the face rest is completely out of the way.

Skirts should not be an issue as long as your chair does not have a support bar that comes up between the legs. If a woman is wearing a long narrow skirt, she may need to hike it up a little just to lift the leg over the chair, then the skirt can come down.

Make sure they slide their bum forward in the seat as far as is comfortable. This brings the abdomen against the chest support and ensures that they have good support for their back. If they don't get forward right from the beginning, they'll slide forward as you go through your massage and this will throw off the positioning of their neck and head in the face rest as they settle into the chair.

Get them to put their shins on the shin rests before they lean forward. Ask if their knees are comfortable in that position.

Support for the torso...

Ask them to lean forward onto the chest support and put their arms on the armrest. If your chest support is adjustable, it's important that you lock it in place before they lean forward. If it's not, they'll push the lower end of the chest support forward into a vertical position and lose any abdominal support.

Get them to relax forward completely onto the support. Some people have a tendency to hold themselves a little rigid. Use some imagery to help them relax. Try phrases like:

"Let yourself fall onto the chest pad"

"Drop into the chest support"

"Relax completely into this chest pad"

If you need to, gently stroke from the center of their back out to their shoulders as a tactile cue to let the shoulders fall forward.

Once they've relaxed forward, it's time to do a quick visual inspection of their position in the chair.

- Make sure that their lower back looks relatively flat and is not swaying forward.

- Check to see that there is no space between their body and the chest pad; that their body is completely relaxed forward.

- Look to see that the chest pad is approximately in the center of their torso. It should cover both their navel and their nipples.

If anything looks amiss, then get them to sit upright, make any adjustments you need to make to the chest support or the pad and then repeat the visual scan. Ask them if they are comfortable.

The tricky part...

The face rest is the trickiest part of the chair to adjust properly. It takes a lot of practice to get it right.

You want to accomplish two things with the face rest adjustment.

1. You want to get their neck into a comfortable flexed position. If their neck is extended at all, they are going to become very uncomfortable in the chair. Avoid extension in the neck as much as possible.

2. You want to get very even support around the whole face so that no particular part of the face bears the weight of the head.

I want to emphasize again as you begin to set up their face in the face cradle, that the face rest should be down so that they don't automatically aim their head for the hole.

Once they are relaxed on the chest support and you've done your visual scan, then come to the front of the chair and loosen all adjustments on the face rest if possible. Start with the face rest in the lowest possible position.

To get their neck in a comfortable flexed position, ask them to drop their head forward slightly or to drop their chin to their chest. Watch that they don't jut their chin forward and put their neck into extension. If necessary, use a hand to guide their head into the desired position, just like a hairstylist does when cutting your hair. Ask them to hold that position. Your aim is to get their neck slightly flexed.

Why is it important to get their neck flexed? If you take a look at the illustration below, you'll see the neck in both an extended and flexed position. When the neck is extended, the small joints at the back of the vertebrae, called the *facet joints*, move closer together and become compressed. If this position is maintained for any length of time, the neck starts to feel achy. When the head is flexed forward, however, the facet joints are separated. This "opened" or lengthened position of the neck is very comfortable.

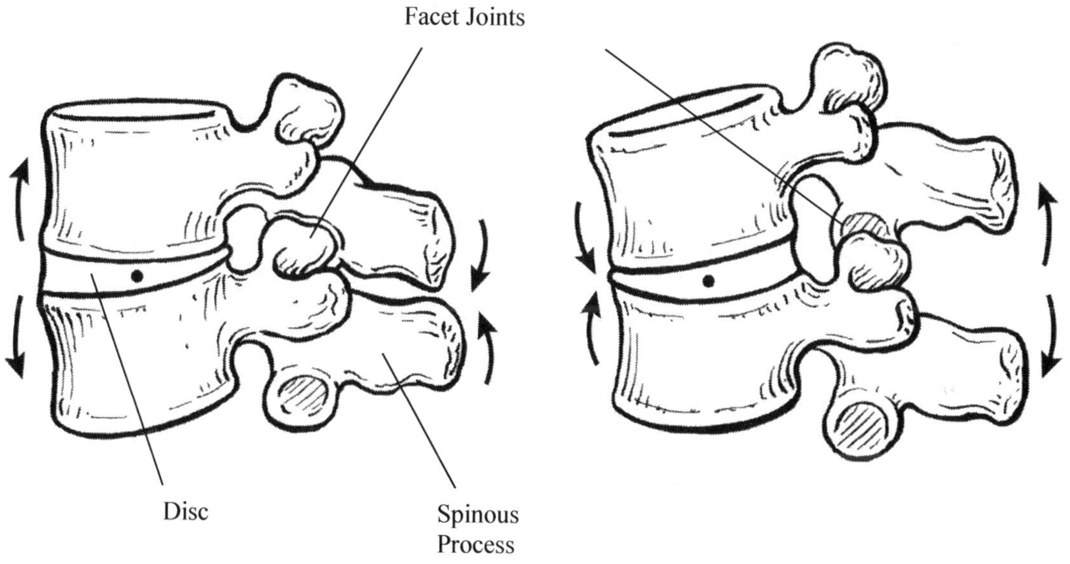

Facet Joints

Disc

Spinous
Process

What you are going to do next is bring the face rest up to meet their face as they stay in that flexed position. To do this, stand upright in front of the chair and hold the lower part of the face rest with two hands. You want to be able to support the weight of the head if they let their full weight fall into the cradle. By holding the bottom ends of the face rest, you have more control over the double action. If you hold to close to the top of the face rest, you'll find that you won't be able to control the forward translation of the face rest; you'll only be able to utilize the tilt function.

Standing upright also allows you to see that their head is positioned properly in the hole and that their neck remains in a nicely flexed position. Don't try to see their face through the hole. If you squat down to do this, you'll lose the visual sense of their positioning and you won't be able to properly support the face rest.

Notice the plane of their face and adjust the tilt of the face rest to match that angle. Keeping the face rest on that plane, simply lift the face rest to meet their face. As you do this, imagine the seam at the top of the hole coming above their eyebrows.

This is where the biggest mistake is made in adjusting the face rest. The practitioner imagines the nose as a dart going for the bull's-eye at the center of a target. In this case, the target is the face pad. If you do this, you'll find that the person's face will be positioned too high in the face rest and their eyes will be squished on the top edge of the pad.

Think of the eyes as being in the center of their face. Direct the face rest so that the widest part of the hole (the center of the pad) is at the same level as their eyes.

I can't emphasize enough the importance of making this adjustment properly. Not only does it make them more comfortable in the chair, but it will also prevent them from fainting.

Stop them from fainting...

Fainting episodes with chair massage is a common occurrence. We've discussed this phenomenon when we discussed *Side Effects*.

You can largely stop this from happening by adjusting the face rest properly. When the face is positioned too high on the face rest, the ends of the face pad will rest against the front of the neck. This puts pressure on the carotid sinuses, which can cause a very rapid reflex drop in blood pressure.

So you need to position the face rest relatively high on their face, so that the lower ends of the face pad come against the jaw and not the neck.

Once you have the face rest positioned where you think it needs to go, ask them to let the weight of their head drop fully into the face cradle. Be sure to stabilize it in that position. Use both hands to hold the face rest and if necessary, put your body against it to hold it in place. Then ask the person to lift their head for a moment. Watching not to move the face rest, lock it into position. Instruct the person to drop their face back into the rest.

Now we can step back and do a visual scan of the neck:

- Check to see that the neck is slightly flexed. The cervical spine should appear flat.

- Look to see that there is some clearance between the bottom ends of the face pad and their neck.

- Look up through the hole in the face rest to make sure their eyes are positioned across the widest part of the hole.

Many people have a "head forward carriage" that results in some structural hyperlordosis (excessive curvature) of their neck. You'll notice this visually as you are talking to your customer. Their head doesn't sit over their body i.e. the ears over the shoulders, but is pulled forward, well in front of their center of gravity.

When you see someone with this kind of head carriage, it is unlikely that you will be able to flatten out the curve by flexing their head forward. In these cases, the bony and connective tissue structures have adapted to this position and they will feel comfortable even if the neck appears to be a little extended over a few spinal segments.

Also be aware that people's heads have different widths. If someone's face looks particularly squished or if someone's face is falling through the hole, you can usually detach the ends of the face pad and move them closer together or further apart to make the individual comfortable.

When you've finished setting up the face rest, just check in with your customer to make sure that they feel comfortable before you begin the massage.

Customer set up checklist...

As a summary, here's a brief checklist to get someone set up in the chair:

- ❑ Have the chair in neutral position

- ❑ Demonstrate and describe how to get into the chair (after your screening)

- ❑ Talk the person through the first part of the set up:

  1. "Have a seat"

  2. "Slide forward on the seat"

  3. "Put your legs on the shin rests"

  4. "Let your body fall onto the chest support"

  5. "Your arms go up on the arm rest"

- ❑ Do a visual scan to make sure the back is well supported

- ❑ Ask the person to drop their head forward slightly

- ❑ Bring the face rest up to meet the face

- ❑ Lock the face rest into position

- ❑ Do a visual scan focusing on neck

  1. The cushion should not press into the front of the neck

  2. The neck should not be extended

  3. You should be able to see their eyes through the face rest hole

8 Principles for Efficient Body Use

Chair massage doesn't have to be hard on your body. Stick to these eight body use principles and doing chair massage will be easy and stress free.

I hear a couple of common negative comments about chair massage. One is that the chair massage is really hard on your body. The second is that chair massage is, to quote one professional, "a lot of airy-fairy light touching (which does nothing for the likes of me because I specialize in deep tissue.)"

I'd like to dispel both these myths.

People who find chair massage hard to perform haven't realized that massage done in the chair requires a totally different approach to that done on a table. Chair massage is only hard on your body when you do it wrong. As a practitioner you should look and feel relaxed and comfortable. There is no reason why the average practitioner can't do five or six hours of massage per day.

Using the approach taught at Relax to the Max, you'll find that there is very little stress to your hands and in particular, very little stress to the small joints in your fingers and thumbs. We've specifically designed techniques that avoid the use of these parts of the hand so that you can massage without injury. Instead of doing "thumb circles" for example, we take the unorthodox approach of using the pisiform.

If the massage is airy-fairy or just looks that way, it's because the person using the chair hasn't learned to leverage their body properly or use their body weight effectively. By virtue of your positioning, you can really utilize your weight to advantage. Even small people can feel pretty big when using these techniques. We often get comments from customers that it feels much more effective than the light massage they get on a table.

I'm not suggesting that you should beat up your customers, but you should be aware that chair massage can be as "deep" as you want to make it.

To ensure that you're using your body weight in the best way possible, we utilize a number of body use principles – eight of them to be exact. These underlying principles will assist you in using your body efficiently so that you get the maximum results with the least possible fatigue and stress to your body. Massage is *physical work,* but if proper body mechanics are used it should not be *hard work.*

These principles may seem a little abstract as you read about them, but you will appreciate their value when you see how they apply to your hands-on work. I would highly suggest the companion DVD set that accompanies this book to really get a grasp on these principles.

1. Keep your spine in a neutral alignment

The spine should be held in a neutral position. The curves of the spine should not be exaggerated or minimized. By maintaining this position, your low back is stabilized. In addition, weight and gravity are transferred through the muscles and joints in a balanced manner, which prevents undue strain on your muscles and joints.

Because we generally have sedentary lifestyles, we tend to lack the strength and awareness needed to stabilize the trunk in this neutral position. For this reason you have to be very conscious of holding the spine in this neutral alignment, especially with techniques that involve the transfer of the weight through your arms.

You need to lunge when doing many of the techniques. If our spine is straight in a lunge position, you can see from the illustration that you are looking downward at the floor (fig XXX).

This is a very unnatural position. We have a very instinctive reflex that makes us want to orient our eyes to the horizon. So your natural inclination will be to lift your torso to see straight forward. As you can see from Figure XXX, this takes the back out of a neutral position and causes hyperlordosis (excessive curving) in the low back. This makes it all the more difficult to stabilize the low back and causes undue stress to the spinal joints.

It's important to fight this instinct and to maintain a very neutral position of the spine.

2. Align body segments in the direction of force

Bones and joints of the arm should be lined up in the direction of movement. The pelvis should also be lined up in the direction of the movement. This allows your weight and force to be effectively transferred through your skeletal structure (the bones) and prevents undue strain to the joints, ligaments or muscles. When the direction of movement changes, your whole body must be adjusted to this new direction.

As an example of this, make a loose fist and put your thumb on top of your index finger. Notice how your thumb is lined up along the line of the radius bone. Now push against the tip of your thumb as illustrated in Figure XXX. You can see that there is very little movement in the thumb. And you can feel that there is very little stress on the thumb joints.

To contrast that stable aligned position, lift your thumb off your index finger so that it is more or less at right angles to your forearm. It's no longer in a straight line with your radius bone, but curves away from the arm. Now push against the pad of the thumb. (See figure XXX.) The thumb is more difficult to stabilize and you can see how it moves to accommodate the force. If you press firmly, you can see and feel the stress that is placed on the metacarpal phalangeal joint (where your thumb meets your hand).

In the first position where the segments are aligned in the direction of force, the weight is safely transferred through the bones. In the second position, where the thumb is not aligned in the direction of force, the ligaments around the thumb joints and the muscles at the base of the thumb are subjected to a great deal of strain.

3. Place peripheral joints in a midrange position

The joints should be positioned in midrange, that is, halfway between the extremes of movement for that joint. The joint surfaces will have the broadest possible contact with each

115

other and the joint becomes more stable. And to a certain extent, the muscles can generate more force when the joint is in this position. This decreases the level of required muscular effort.

Always avoid putting the joint in any extreme position, (i.e. hyperextended or hyperflexed).

4. Let your body weight fall forward

For the compression techniques and many of the kneading techniques, you can increase your pressure with minimal effort if you mobilize our body weight to produce the force. When you use the arms and hands alone, a greater amount of effort is exerted to obtain the same level of force.

To transfer your weight effectively the spine needs to be aligned and stabilized and the joints need to be correctly positioned and aligned. One leg will be positioned in front of the other in a lunge position. The front foot and knee are pointed in the direction of the movement. Then simply let your body weight fall into the contact point, that is, the part of your hand or arm that you use for the technique. It's just like you are comfortably leaning against a table or wall. By doing this, you are transferring your body weight safely and effectively through your bones and joints. Little muscular effort is used.

When you are in the lunge position, your weight should always be supported by the front leg. In this way, very little movement is needed to let your weight or centre of gravity fall forward onto the customer. If most of your weight is on the back leg, you need to make a huge shift to get your weight onto the customer.

If you have your weight on your back leg, it's most likely that you won't transfer the weight forward at all. Instead, you will try to generate the force from your upper body and use a lot of muscular effort.

When doing techniques that involve this transfer of body weight, the front knee will always be bent and the back leg will always be straight. Don't let the front knee go forward past the foot when lunging. This puts excessive stress on the knees. And don't try to keep the back foot facing forward. The toes will naturally be directed outward. This will make your stance more stable.

5. Move to maintain good alignment

The techniques are not static and isolated to one area. Rather, you are constantly moving from one region to another. You need to move and adjust your body in order to effectively execute the first four principles. If you do not adjust your distance and remain stationary, you end up reaching and bending because you are too far, or shrugging and stretching because you are too close, or twisting because the contact point is to the side.

So adjust yourself as needed to maintain neutral alignment of the spine, to keep your segments lined up in the direction of force, to place your joints in a mid-range position and to be in a position where you can let your weight fall forward.

6. Use large muscle groups

When applying the techniques, the movement should come from the large muscle groups as opposed to the smaller muscles. For example, when you are doing a circular kneading action with your thumbs, you will stabilize your thumbs in a good alignment with the forearm and use your shoulder muscles to make the movement happen. This is in contrast to using the smaller muscles at the base of your thumb like tiny windshield wipers to create the circular action.

The larger muscle groups can generate more power and will fatigue less easily. The smaller muscles do not have the strength or energy reserve to generate the ongoing force and power necessary to apply hours of massage. They quickly become fatigued and are predisposed to injury.

If you take the Relax to the Max chair massage training, you'll notice that it's your legs and bum that are sore after the first day or two, not your hands or arms.

7. Reinforce your contact point

Reinforce your fingers and thumbs whenever possible. Reinforce the most distal segment.

These smaller joints are more likely to become strained or injured, so support them as much as you can. For example, if you put one thumb on top of the other as you perform a kneading movement, each thumb is doing just half the work. (See Figure XXX.) To look at it another way, with your thumbs reinforced, you can apply twice as much pressure as you could with just one thumb.

8. Integrate a relaxation phase into each techniques

Each technique has a work phase and a release phase. In other words, you are only expending energy through part of each technique. If you don't allow your muscle to go through that release phase, your muscles will remain contracted. When a muscle contracts it uses more oxygen and nutrients, but at the same time it squeezes off its own blood supply. Thus, the muscle runs out of oxygen and waste products accumulate. The muscle fatigues and starts to ache. However, when you allow for a relaxation phase, the muscle is able to relax. Carbon dioxide and wastes are flushed out of the muscle and oxygen and nutrients are replenished.

With some techniques, like simple compressions, the relaxation occurs when you lift your hand to move to the next position. With other techniques, like kneading, you don't break contact and you have to be more consciously aware of relaxing your arm though part of the movement.

Techniques

At last, we can start massaging. In the following sections you'll learn a wide variety of techniques that cover your customer from head to toe. We'll teach you the special 15-minute routine developed by Relax to the Max. Then we'll look at a range of additional techniques, including ones to the lower body. By the end of this section you'll be able to customize your massage to meet your customers' needs, whether it's a 2-minute test drive or a one-hour full body massage done right in the chair.

The techniques you'll learn in this book have been developed through market testing. We did research with a large group of people to come up with the most advantageous techniques. We gave each person a massage using both Swedish and Shiatsu style techniques as well as some unique techniques that were designed specifically for the chair.

After each massage we asked the person to tell us which techniques they enjoyed the most and which ones they liked least. We continued with this process, dropping the techniques people didn't like and keeping the ones they did. Our only criterion was that the techniques feel terrific. By the end, we had an arsenal of techniques that had universal appeal – everybody loved them.

From those techniques we chose the ones that were easiest on your body as a practitioner. These are the techniques you learn in the program. We are not faithful to any particular school of bodywork or massage. Our primary criteria in choosing techniques for the course were that the techniques were enjoyable and safe for the customer and placed a minimal amount of stress on the practitioner's body.

In the following pages, you will find a variety of Shiatsu (acupressure) and Swedish style techniques as well as techniques that were designed specifically to take advantage of the unique features of the chair.

Categorizing the techniques

In general, the techniques can be broken into several broad categories: compression techniques, kneading techniques, squeezing techniques and percussion techniques.

Compression techniques are like many Shiatsu techniques. They involve a straight compression into the tissue with some part of your body, like your thumb or elbow for example. The most important element to remember when performing any compression technique is that **the pressure is applied at right angles** (at 90 degrees or perpendicular) to the area of the body being worked on.

Kneading techniques involve a circular motion. Remember as you are doing kneading actions to **relax through part of each movement**. When doing compression or squeezing techniques, you have to relax your hands as you lift them to move to another area. With kneading techniques, this release phase is not inherent in the movement. So you need to make a conscious effort to do so or else your hands and your body will fatigue quickly.

Squeezing techniques are just as the name implies: A muscle is squeezed between two contact points. The most important thing to remember when performing any squeezing technique is to **get your contact points on the edge of the muscle**. Grab too little and you'll pinch your customer, grab too much and you will likely be squeezing bones.

Percussion techniques are old Swedish-style techniques in which light springy blows are applied to the body. They tend to be invigorating.

Other notes

Add a preface along these lines:

There's method to our madness. The application of the techniques is very methodical. We do things in a certain way for good reason. Very little happens by accident.

It's difficult to go through our entire rationale for doing the techniques the way we do. That kind of information is contained in our teacher's manual and is a book on its own. What is presented here is a cursory description. We encourage you to view the accompanying videotapes or better yet attend a class.

Learning massage is like learning a sport. It's one thing to read about, but another thing entirely to do it. It's a physical skill and there is no replacement for an experienced coach who can examine your body use, analyze your approach and give you constructive feedback to improve. Nothing replaces hands-on learning.

Contact points

Very little of what I (or my instructors) say or do in teaching these chair massage techniques is random. We are very systematic and purposeful in our approach and the language that we use. As you read through descriptions of the various techniques, you should pay close attention to the specific terminology we use in describing the various contact points on your hands and arms. Let me outline some of these for you:

Pads of the fingers: This is the broad surface of the fingers. When you use the pads of your fingers, think of leaving your fingerprints on your customer.

Tips of the fingers: This is the distal ends of the fingers and is much more specific than the pads of the fingers. You'll use the tips of the fingers when you want to catch the edge of a relatively small muscle.

Heel of the hand: The broad part of the hand just distal to the crease of the wrist.

Heel of the thumb: To get technical, the thenar eminence – to be more specific, the metacarpal of the thumb.

Base of the thumb: The head of the metacarpal of the thumb. You'll use this when squeezing small muscles with the hand.

Fist: This is a broad contact with the back of the fist, that is, the flat surfaces of the first phalanges.

Knuckles: These are your big knuckles – your metacarpal phalangeal (MCP) joints. This is in contrast to your proximal interphalangeal joints (your PIP joints) or your distal interphalangeal joints (your DIP joints).

Elbow: The olecranon process, that is, the pointy part of your elbow. To use a specific point like this, the elbow is usually quite flexed.

Open elbow: To create a broader contact, you can extend the elbow slightly so that the contact is not directly on the olecranon, but along the proximal ulna. This is a very distinct boney ridge.

As a general rule, when you want the massage to feel deeper or more penetrating, you'll use a small contact point. Why? Because you have the same force going through a smaller area, you are increasing the pressure (pounds per square inch).

The opposite is also true. If someone is particularly sensitive, then use a broader contact so that the force is dispersed over a wider area.

Routine Techniques

We refer to the first techniques we'll cover as the "routine techniques". At Relax to the Max these particular techniques are used in a standardized 15-minute massage routine. Essentially, we took a number of the techniques that we developed through our market testing and used them to create a comprehensive sequence for use in the corporate environment. We experimented with the technique selection, the sequencing and the pacing until we got it just right. This is a routine that we have refined to perfection over the past ten years.

Because this particular sequence was developed for the corporate market, it was designed to be relaxing, but at the same time invigorating. In surveys I've done for corporations, I measured the employees' subjective responses to this massage in a number of different areas. In a compilation of surveys taken over a one-year period of office workers who received this routine massage, 99% reported that they felt more relaxed and 97% felt less tension. At the same time, however, the majority or 94% said they felt more clearheaded after the massage and 89% reported feeling energized.

I like using a routine like this one for a number of reasons.

1. For me, a standardized routine has ensured a consistent quality of massage. For example, I've brokered some large jobs where I've had 25 practitioners working at the same time on a large group of people. In those kinds of situations where a number of practitioners are working together, you want to ensure that every customer receives the same level of quality. A standardized routine with consistent techniques, timing, and pacing guarantees that will happen.

2. In doing chair massage, you'll find yourself in environments where there are often lots of distractions – tradeshows, festivals, events, etc. You don't want to find yourself in the situation where you get half way through a massage and forget whether you've massaged both sides of the body or whether you've just done the one side. When you use a routine, the sequence becomes very automatic, almost like driving a car. Your massage won't be ruined by distractions. If you are doing technique A, then you know that technique B comes next. It's as simple as that.

3. Lastly, the routine serves as a skeleton or a framework that you can build upon as your skills develop. I've trained in classical ballet and I can tell you that whether you've danced for one year or 40 years you always start with the same basic exercises at the beginning of each class. This is true of many disciplines. I was told by a karate black belt that you don't get proficient by doing 1,000 things, but by

doing the same thing 1,000 times. Get good at a routine and then build onto it as your skill level grows.

> "For a long time I limited myself to one color – as a form of discipline."
> – *Pablo Picasso on his Blue and Rose periods*

Okay! Let's get started. We'll start by looking at the techniques that we use as the basis of the standardized 15-minute routine at Relax to the Max. They are listed in the order in which they occur in the routine.

At the end of this section you'll find the outline of the routine. We highly suggest getting the Chair Massage Techniques DVD to help you understand these techniques and the routine on a deeper level.

1. Gentle circles

Position and body use

- Begin by standing to one side of your partner to work on the opposite side of the back

- Don't bend forward from the waist. Take a nice wide lunge position to keep your back aligned

Performing the technique

- Using your heel of your hand, do gentle circles over the erector spinae

- Move your circles from the top of the back to the top the hips, overlapping the circles with each repetition

- If you find yourself stooping or bending to reach your partner's back, widen your stance

Other tips

- Don't apply any significant pressure. This technique is not done to manipulate the muscles, but rather to simply give the person a chance to settle into the chair and relax. Think of this technique as a shirt massage, rather than a muscle massage.

- Even though the heel of the hand is the contact point, let the entire hand rest comfortably on the back.

- Make the circles large enough that the customer can differentiate sensations, but not so wide as to feel as if they are being groped.

2. Trap squeeze

Position and body use
- Stand behind your partner and drape your hands over your partner's shoulders. The heel of your hand will rest on the back edge of the traps and your fingertips will rest on the front edge of the upper traps

- Keep your shoulders relaxed

- It may be useful to use a pincer palpation to find the edge of the muscle before performing the squeezes

Performing the technique
- Gently squeeze the muscle between the heel of your hand and your fingertips

- Begin the squeezes at the neck-shoulder junction and then shift laterally after each squeeze

- Near the neck, you'll find that you'll do the compression more between the heel of your thumb and your first two fingers. As you move lateral, it will be easier to use the whole heel of the hand

Other tips
- It is important that you are able to define the borders of the muscle

- If your fingertips are placed too far in front of the anterior edge of the trapezius, you'll pull the skin taut against the front of the throat and your customer will feel as if they are being choked. If your fingers are too much on top of the trapezius, you'll end up pinching their skin

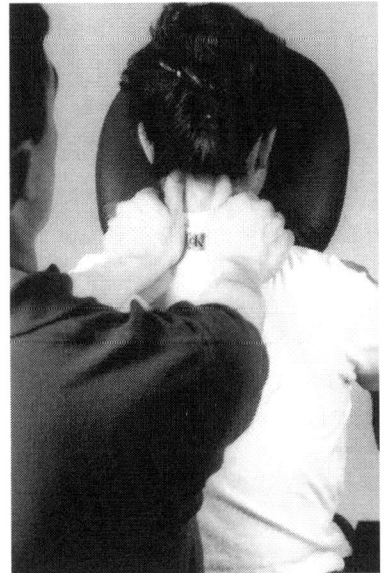

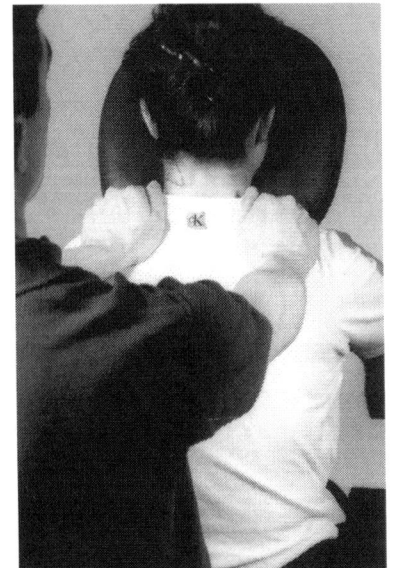

126

- Likewise, make sure that the heels of the hand are far enough down the back

- Keep the thumbs tucked into the hand to prevent stress to those joints

Note: An alternative to the trap squeeze is performed by squeezing and then gently shaking the muscle back and forth several times with a loose easy movement while maintaining the squeeze.

3. Butterfly

Position and body use

- Get into a lunge position behind your partner

- Place the heels of your thumbs directly beside the spinous processes with the thumbs pointing straight up

- As you do this technique down the back, you'll need to move your back foot further away from the chair with each subsequent repetition to maintain a neutral alignment of your spine.

Performing the technique

- With your elbows only slightly bent, slowly let your weight fall into your hands

- Do this by lifting the front leg off the floor

- Place the front foot back on the floor to slowly release the pressure

- Slide the hands down several inches and repeat the compression

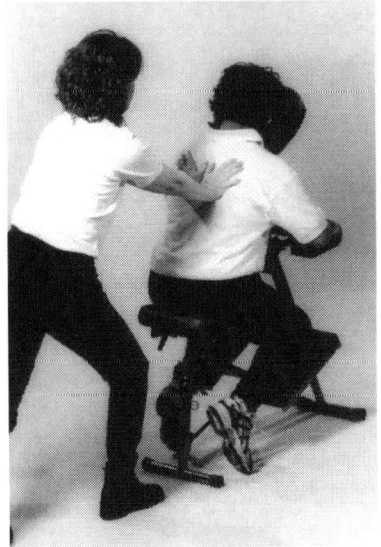

Other tips

- Once you get a sense for transferring your weight through your arms, you no longer will need to lift the front leg

- Be sure to stabilize the elbows and shoulders so that no movement occurs in your arms

- Likewise be sure stabilize the trunk so that you neither extend nor flex your low back

- Keep your center of gravity low to prevent excessive flexion of the wrists

- If you get even the slightest discomfort in your wrist use the alternative Fist Compression technique

The upper back is usually too horizontal to let your weight fall forward effectively, so you'll likely need to use the strength in your arm muscles to do the compression for the first two or three compressions

4. Pisiform circles to the erectors

Position and body use

- Stand in a lunge behind your partner and slightly off to one side

- If you are massaging the right side of the back, stand slightly to the left and use your right hand to perform the technique

- To find the starting position for the pisiform, place the pisiform bone of the right hand on the crest of the erector spinae, about one inch lateral to the spinous processes on the right side of your partner's back.

- Then move the skin and the material of the shirt medial and inferior so that the pisiform is sitting in the laminar groove

- By doing this, you have some additional slack in the skin so that you can perform the technique across the whole width of the muscle

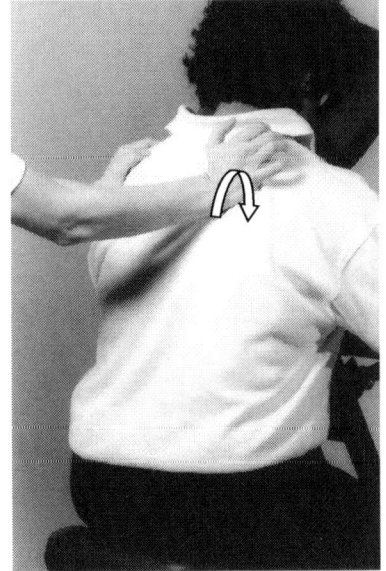

Performing the technique

- Start at about the C7 level

- Stabilize your arm and your trunk Let your weight fall through the pisiform and allow it to move upwards and outwards across the muscle

- Release the pressure but keep the contact as you bring the skin and shirt back to the starting position to complete the circle

- Repeat the circle several times in the one spot, lift and move the pisiform down the back a few inches and repeat the technique

Other tips

- The skin and shirt material must move with the hand throughout the movement. Do not glide over the material.

- Don't lift the fingers or extend the wrist. Keep the palm facing the back and let your fingers relax.

- Be careful not to do the movement with your arm and shoulder. Your trunk and arm are stabilized and you simply transfer your body weight by rocking your body back and forth.

If you feel a strong strumming sensation, you are pushing directly across the muscle. To correct this, stand more behind your partner and think of your pisiform moving UP along the medial edge of the erector spinae rather than ACROSS. Your "circles" become tall ovals.

5. Elbow compressions to the mid-back

Position and body use

- Stand behind and slightly to the side of your partner

- Your hips are facing straight forward

- If you are massaging the right side of the back, your right leg comes forward beside your partner and your left hip is directly behind your partner's spine

- Use the elbow closest to your partner, in this case the left elbow

- Don't flex the elbow sharply. Keep it relatively open or extended

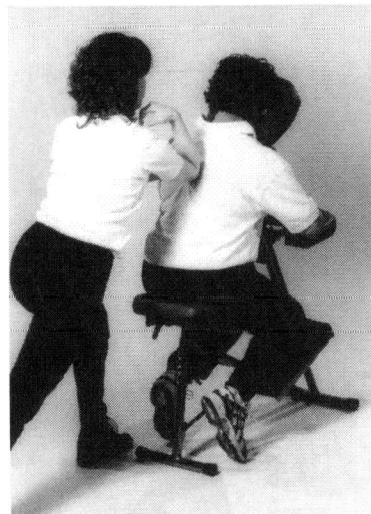

Performing the technique

- Place the elbow in the laminar groove near C7, slowly let your weight fall forward into the elbow, hold and release

- Slide down a couple of inches to the next position and repeat the compression

- Once you reach the mid-back (around the bra line), lift the elbow and place it on the crest of the erector spinae at the C7 level

- Perform a series of compressions down the crest of the erector spinae to the mid-back

- Repeat to the left side

Other tips

- It is extremely important that you move the back leg backwards slightly after each compression to maintain the neutral alignment of your spine

- Because your elbow is so close to the spinous processes, it is important that you shoulder is directly behind your elbow and that you direct your pressure anterior. If you are positioned on an oblique angle, your elbow will push into the spinous processes.

- To disperse your force, open up the elbow so that your weight is spread out along the ridge of the ulna. For a more penetrating technique, flex the elbow sharply and contact with the point of the elbow.

- If using the point of the elbow, cup your elbow with your free hand to provide support and to prevent slipping (see photo)

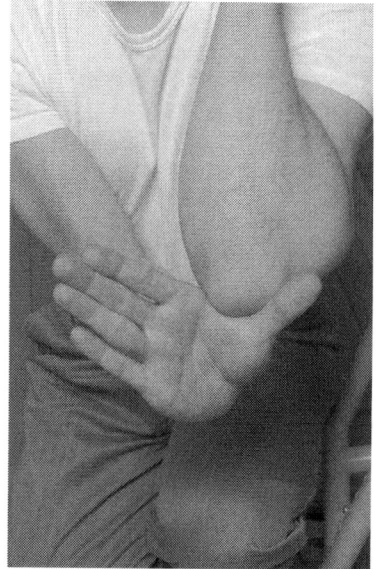

•

6. Deltoid squeeze

Position and body use

- Kneel or squat beside your partner facing their arm

- Interlace your fingers and place the heels of the hands on the edges of the deltoid muscle at the top of the arm

- Keep the heels of the hands aligned vertically along the edges of the muscle

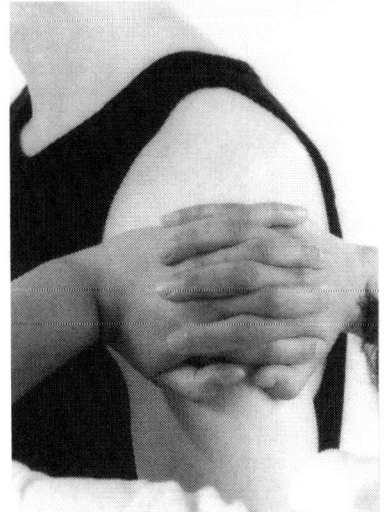

Performing the technique

- Gently compress the edges of the deltoid with the heels of your hands and release

- Move down slightly and repeat

- Continue these squeezes down the length of the deltoid (approximately one third of the way done the upper arm)

Other tips

- Keep the elbows high if possible so that the forearms are parallel to the ground. This will allow you to use your chest muscles to generate force.

- It is difficult to palpate the edges of the deltoid where it inserts into the humerous. Be sure not to go more than a third of the way down the arm or you'll end up pinching the skin and fat on the outside of the arm.

7a. Double arm squeeze

Position and body use

- Kneel or squat beside your partner facing their arm

- Mold one hand to the biceps muscle. The fingers should be pointing away from you so that the heel of the hand is lined up vertically along the edge of the biceps. You thumb should lie along the anterior-inferior edge of the deltoid

- The other hand surrounds the triceps. The side of the index finger can be placed high up in the armpit

- Notice that there's a significant difference in height between the front hand and the back hand, with the bicep hand positioned somewhat lower.

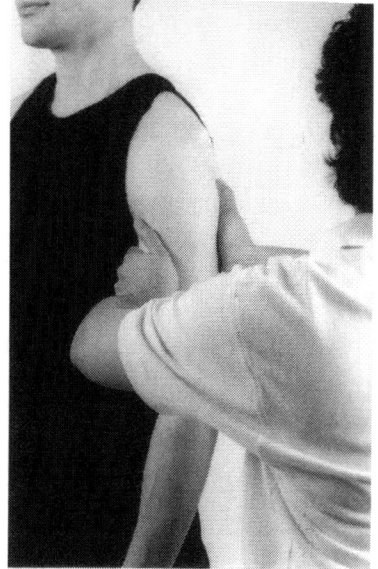

Performing the technique

- Squeeze the muscles between the heel of the hands and the flat surfaces of the fingers as you push your hands gently towards each other

- Release and slide downward slightly

- Repeat the sequence finishing at the elbow

Other tips

- The most significant action is the squeezing between the heel of the hand and the fingers. We have you push your hands together slightly so that your contact points stay on the edges of the muscle. Otherwise, your hands will tend to slide off the muscle, pinching the skin and fat on their arms. This is particularly important if your partner has large upper arms.

- Be careful not to position yourself too closely to your partner. You'll tend to lift the arm

135

upward and will not be able to generate any significant force as you try to push your hands towards each other.

- Because of poor posture, your partner's arms may tend to internally rotate – you'll see the palm facing backwards rather than facing the body. As a result, the biceps are against the body rather than being anterior as they should be if the arm is in a neutral position with the palm facing the body. Be aware of this so that you can grab the muscle itself rather than the skin and fat on the medial and lateral surfaces of the arm. You can use the single-handed biceps or triceps squeeze (as outlined below in 7b and 7c) in place of the double arm squeeze if your partner has smaller arms.

7b. Triceps squeeze

Position and body use

- Kneel, squat or sit beside your partner

- Using the hand that is closest to the front of your partner, take the wrist and lift the arm slightly away from the body

- Mold the other hand to the back of the arm and slide the fingers upward so that they rest under the armpit

Performing the technique

- Squeeze the triceps muscle between the heel of your hand and the flat surface of your fingers

- Release, slide downward and repeat the squeeze

- Continue this pattern until you reach the bottom of the triceps, at the elbow

Other tips

- Use the flat surfaces of your fingers rather than the fingertips, that is, your hand will be in a "V" shape rather than a "C" shape.

- To avoid pinching skin, be sure that your hand goes around the whole width of the muscle. If necessary, place the free hand on the front of the elbow so that you can push forward slightly with the working hand.

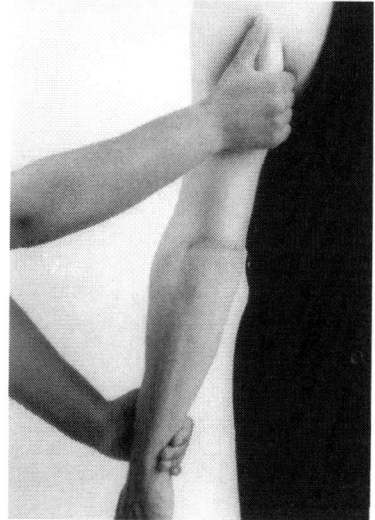

7c. Biceps squeeze

Position and body use
- Kneel, squat or sit beside your partner

- Take your partner's wrist with your other hand and lift the arm away slightly from the body

- Mold the other hand to the front of the arm so that your thumb lies along the front edge of the deltoid muscle

Performing the technique
- Squeeze the biceps muscle between the heel of your hand and the flat surface of your fingers

- Release, slide downward and repeat the squeeze

- Continue this pattern until you reach the bottom of the biceps, at the level of the elbow

Other tips
- As with the triceps squeeze, if your partner has large arms relative to your hands, use your free hand to support the upper arm rather than the wrist

- Use the flat surfaces of your fingers rather than the fingertips, that is, your hand will be in a "V" shape rather than a "C" shape.

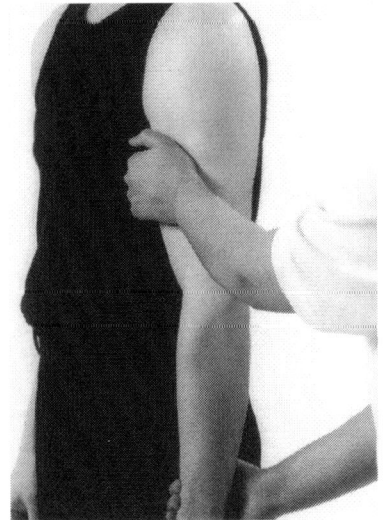

8. Wrist flexor squeeze

Position and body use

- Kneel or squat slightly behind your partner and facing forward in the same direction as your partner

- Using the hand that is furthest from your partner, take the wrist and lift the arm slightly away from the body

- Put the fingertips of the working hand in the cubital fossa (the hollow at the front of the elbow) and the heel of the hand just to the inside of the ulna

Performing the technique

- Squeeze the wrist flexor muscles between the heel of your hand and the tips of your fingers

- Release, slide downwards and repeat the squeeze

- Continue until you reach the bottom of the wrist flexors, just above the wrist

Other tips

- Note that the muscle turns into tendons about two thirds of the way down the forearm. As you squeeze through the lower half of the forearm, you'll see the fingers curl

- Avoid squeezing the forearm bones by keeping your contact points on the edges of the flexors along the whole length of the forearm

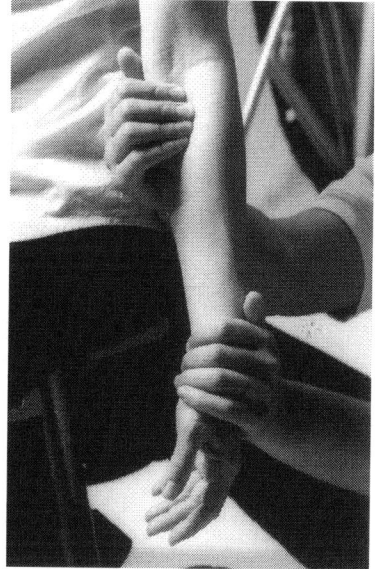

9. Wrist extensor squeeze

Position and body use

- Kneel or squat slightly behind your partner facing forward

- Hold your partner's wrist with the hand that is closest to your partner

- Place the base of your thumb in the hollow behind the elbow and the fingertips in the hollow at the front of the elbow

Performing the technique

- Squeeze the wrist extensor muscles between the base of your thumb and the tips of your fingers

- Release, slide downwards a small distance and repeat the squeeze

- Continue this pattern through the top third of the forearm

Other tips

- The muscles become tendinous about one third of the way down the forearm. There is too little tissue to squeeze below that point.

- Avoid squeezing the bones and be sure to have your contact points on the edge of the muscle

- Because this is a very small muscle group, you'll notice an open space between the palm of your hand and the muscle

- If your hand is positioned correctly, you'll notice that the thumb is oriented upwards, as if you are hitchhiking

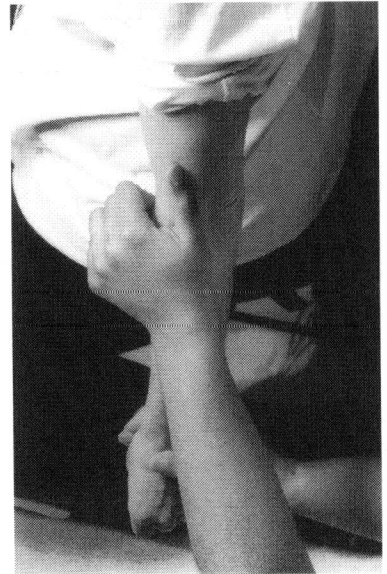

140

10. Pressure points to the palm

Position and body use

- Rest both sets of fingers under the hand

- Use the pads of the thumbs to do compressions along the sides of the metacarpal bones

- Reinforce the thumbs by placing one on top of the other

Performing the technique

- Follow the lines in the attached picture starting at the outside of the base of the small finger

- Do four compressions along each line starting proximal and working distal

- Press in gradually and release the pressure gradually

- On the outside edge of the metacarpal of the thumb, push the muscle to the center of the hand rather than compress downward to avoid pressing directly on the metacarpal bone

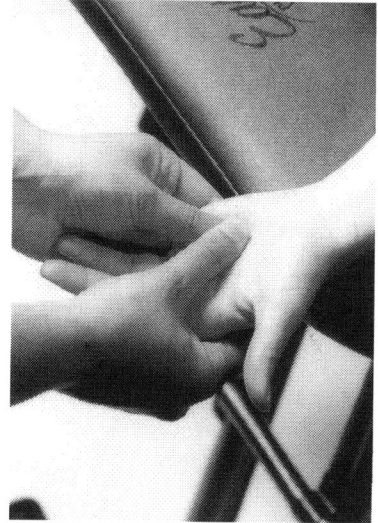

Other tips

- These compressions are intended for the intrinsic muscles of the hand between the metacarpals.

- Be careful not to press directly on either the carpal bones or the metacarpal bones

- Note that there are two lines of compressions between the metacarpals of the thumb and index finger. Line 5 follows the metacarpal of the index finger while Line6 follows along the thumb

11. Shaking the metacarpals

Position and body use
- Grasp the head of the fifth metacarpal between the thumb and index finger of one hand and grasp the head of the fourth metacarpal with the other hand

- Be sure to grab just proximal to the knuckle

- Keep your feet together and position your shoulders directly above your partner's hand

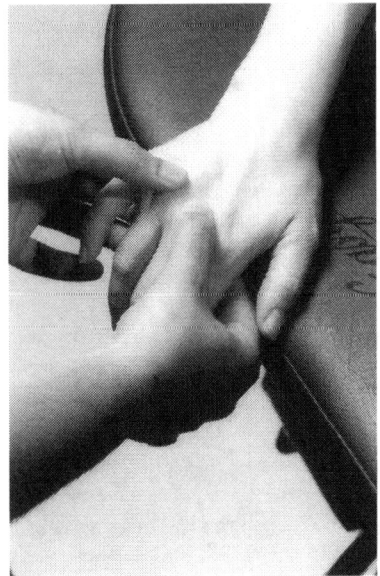

Performing the technique
- Push one metacarpal away as you pull the other toward you and reverse

- Do this at a quick rate so that you are shaking the metacarpals back and forth

- Shift each hand over to the next fingers and repeat to all metacarpals

Other tips
- The aim of this technique is to stretch the intrinsic muscles of the hand

- In order for your partner to feel much sensation, you'll need to be vigorous with the movement

- Keep the elbows relatively straights so that the movement comes from the upper body rather than the elbows or wrists

- Because there is so much movement in the thumb, don't try to push the range of movement

142

12. The "Inch worm"

Position and body use

- Place your partner's hand loosely in yours as if you are shaking hands

- Gently support your partner's hand and extend their wrist

- Place the side of your index finger underneath the base of the little finger

- Place the pad of the thumb on top of the finger while keeping your thumb in line with your partner's finger as illustrated

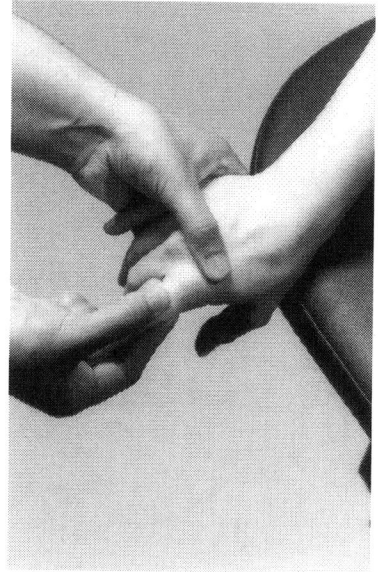

Performing the technique

- Lift your thumb and place it distally a quarter inch

- Push the index finger upwards as it slides distally to meet the thumb (this places a small stretch on the underside of the finger)

- Repeat until you reach the tip of the finger

- Repeat for each finger

Other tips

- The thumb simple stabilizes the finger. Don't slide the thumb proximal as the finger slides distal or you'll pull the skin on top of the finger

- Be careful not to slide your index finger past your thumb or you may push your partner's fingers into hyperextension, which may be uncomfortable

- Be sure to contact with the *side* of the index finger at the DIP joint and avoid using the pad of the finger

- Avoid pulling the finger upward and hyperextending your partner's fingers at the metacarpal-phalangeal joint

13. Dorsal glide

Position and body use

- Put your fingers under your partner's hand and rest the heels of your thumbs on the back of your partner's hand

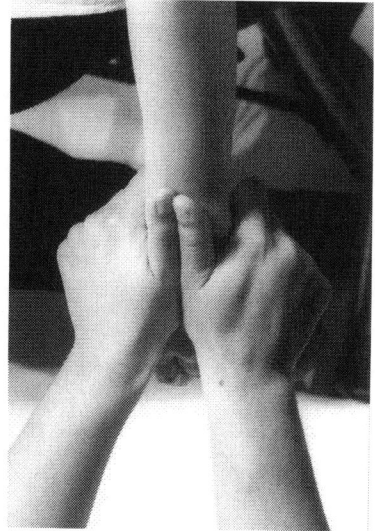

Performing the technique

- Glide the heels of your thumbs outward across the top of your partner's hand in a way that resembles breaking a Popsicle

- Your fingers push gently into the hand and do not slide

Other tips

- Be careful not to use the thumbs themselves. This causes stress to the metacarpal phalangeal (MCP) joint of the thumb

14a. Cat paw

Position and body use
- Stand in front of your partner with feet together

- Place the heel of your hands on top of the shoulders (the crest of the trapezius muscle) as close to the neck as possible

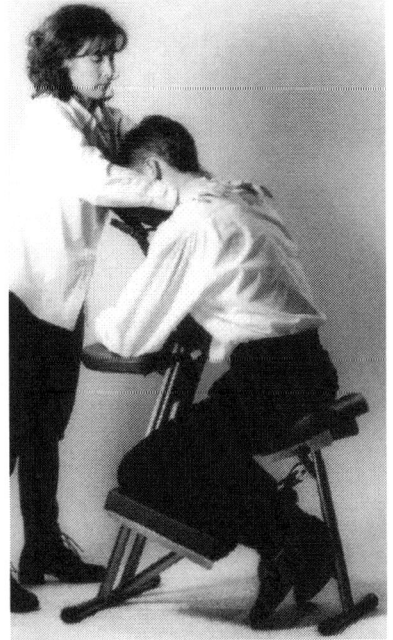

Performing the technique
- Push firmly down into the muscle with one hand directing the pressure to the opposite side of the pelvis

- Push firmly down into the muscle with the second hand and as the other lifts up

- As one hand pushes down the other lifts up in a rhythmical way that resembles a cat pawing the floor

- Move the first hand slightly lateral and repeat the compression

- Work towards the tip of the shoulders with each subsequent compression

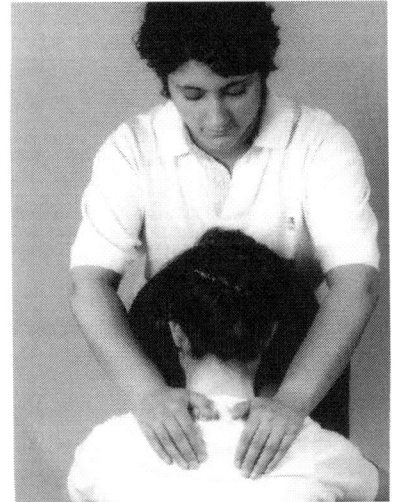

Other tips
- Remember that the hands never lose contact with your partner's shoulders. One hand is always applying pressure or else the movement begins to feel punchy

- Stay on soft tissue and avoid pushing on the clavicle or acromion

- Be careful that the heels of the hands do not drop in front of the traps

146

14b. Cat paw squeeze

Position and body use

- Positioning is the same as the Cat Paw

- Make sure that the heels of the hands are on the crest of the muscle and let the fingers relax down the back

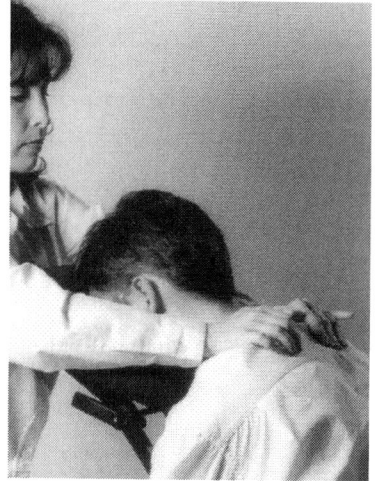

Performing the technique

- The movement is essentially the same the Cat Paw, but a squeezing action is introduced

- As you compress with the heel of the hand, use the pads of your fingers to pull the soft tissue up into the heel of your hand

- Grab as much of the upper-back muscles as possible

- Start close to the neck and work laterally

Other tips

- Don't think of this technique as a trap squeeze performed from the front of the chair. Rather it's a squeeze of the upper back muscles

- To ensure the compression is done at a right angle to the trapezius muscle, the fingers should make a V-position on your partner's back

- Notice in the illustration how the finger joints are extended so that the hand forms a V-shape rather than a C-shape. This allows you to grab more tissue and prevents you from pinching.

15. Elbow pressure points to the traps

Position and body use

- Stand in a lunge position facing your partner and off to one side. Locate the notch on the top edge of the shoulder, where your shoulder blade and collar bone meet (the acromioclavicular notch)

- The hand that is furthest away from your partner's back forms a C-shape and rests on the shoulder, exposing the notch

- Place the elbow so that it is cupped within the "C" of your other hand

Performing the technique

- Let your weight fall forward to gently compress the trapezius

- Direct your pressure towards the opposite side of the pelvis

- Release your pressure and move the elbow and supporting hand medial along the crest of the traps and repeat the compression

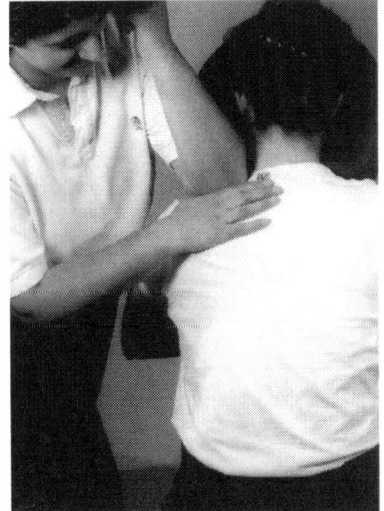

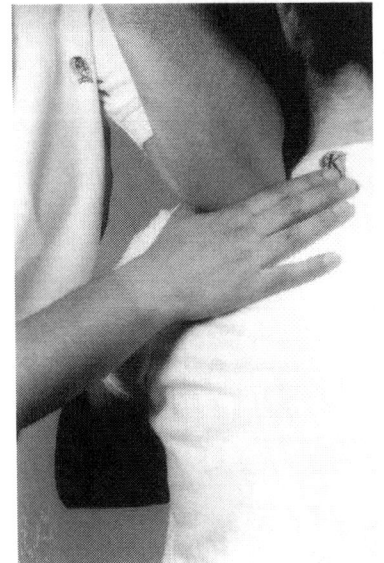

Other tips

- Instead of using the point of the elbow, try opening up the elbow and using the edge of the ulna. It's a broader contact and it removes the possibility of slipping off the crest of the traps.

- If you face your partner head on, your upper arm will bump against their head. To prevent this from happening, swing your back leg away from the chair so that you are at a bit of an angle to your partner.

- As an alternative, this technique can also be done standing behind your partner or beside your partner

16. Thumb compressions beside the edge of the scapula

Position and body use

- Stand behind and slightly to the side of your partner in a lunge position

- Be sure to keep your thumbs lined up in a straight line with your forearms

- Locate the top corner (superior angle) of the shoulder blade and place your reinforced thumbs below this point just medial to the edge of the shoulder blade

Performing the technique

- With your elbows slightly bent, lean your body weight into your thumbs to compress

- Slide your thumbs down and repeat the sequence about two thirds of the way down the shoulder blade

- Do not push against the scapula itself, rather, direct the pressure into the tendons that attach into the shoulder blade

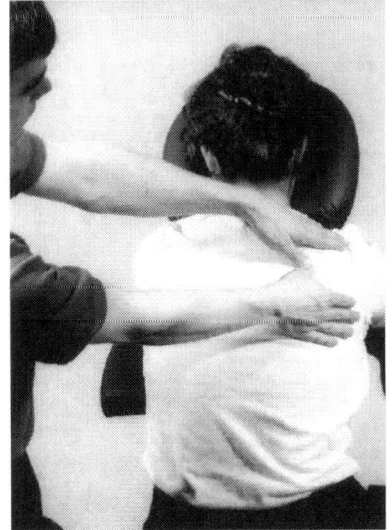

Other tips

- As with all compression techniques, if you are transferring your weight effectively there should be no movement in your body

- There is a tendency to let the palms lie flat on the back and this takes the thumbs out of alignment. Use your fingers as a tripod to keep your palms away from the body (as illustrated), or simply tuck the fingers in to make loose open fists

- If you have hypermobile thumb joints, use one of the alternative techniques that will be presented later to prevent undue stress to your thumb

17. C-scoops

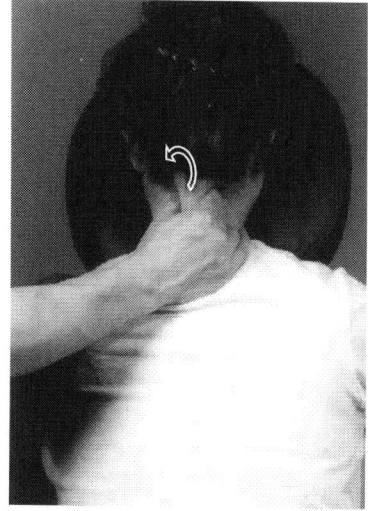

Position and body use

- Stand beside your partner facing forward and with your feet together

- Place your open hand (a C-shape) across the neck just below the base of the skull

- Place the fingertips and the thumb on the lateral edges of the extensor muscles

- To create some slack in the skin, move the skin downward slightly toward the front of the throat

Performing the technique

- From this starting position, lift the neck extensors up along the length of the neck and then away from the neck in a circular pattern, much like lifting a cat by the scruff of the neck

- Clamp the extensor muscles of the neck as your hand move up and away from the body

- Don't slide on the skin. Be sure to move the skin with your fingers

- Release the pressure as you complete a circle to go back to the starting position

- Repeat several times, then place the hand a little lower on the neck to repeat again

Other tips

- These movements should be big, round and rhythmical.

- Emphasize pulling away from the neck (like picking up a cat) and don't push the neck forward into extension

- Be sure to use the tips of the fingers and thumb so that you can catch the edges of the extensors and put a little pull on them

18. Compressions to the base of the skull

Position and body use

- Get into a lunge, slightly to the side of your partner

- If you are working on the right side, you'll stand to the right of your partner with your right leg forward

- Place your reinforced thumbs just to the side of the spinous processes just below the base of the skull

- Make sure the lunge is deep and the elbows are dropped so that the force is directed slightly upward

- Keep your thumbs in the same line as the forearm with one thumb directly on top of the other

Performing the technique

- Gently let the weight fall into the soft tissue below the base of the skull, hold the compression and release

- Repeat a number of times moving laterally across the skull

- Lift your thumbs to change positions and do not slide

Other tips

- This is typically a very tender area so apply the compression slowly and hold it momentarily before releasing

- Push into the soft tissue and not into the skull bone itself

- The base of the skull slopes downward slightly as you move lateral. Don't do a line of compressions straight across or your end up pushing on the skull bone

- Compression techniques are done at right angles to the body. Since the head is round, you'll need to adjust your body position to maintain the 90-degree direction of force. You can do this by swinging the back leg around to the outside

19. Thumb circles to the base of the skull

Position and body use
- Assume the same orientation and stance as you did with the thumb compressions

- To create some slack in the skin, move the skin downward and lateral before beginning the circles. This slack will allow you to make larger circles

Performing the technique
- Let you weight fall forward slightly as the thumb comes up toward the base of the skull in a circular motion

- Moving the skin and the hair with your thumb press upwards and outwards in a half circle

- As your thumbs contact the base of the skull relax the pressure and complete the circle

- Repeat this circular movement three times

- Perform five sets moving laterally under the skull

Other tips
- Lift your thumbs to change positions and do not slide

- Again, the base of the skull angles downward as you move laterally. Be sure to position your thumbs correctly for each set.

- Like the compressions, you'll need to adjust the direction of your force as you continue around the skull

Avoid any sliding. Move the skin and the hair with your thumbs

20. Percussion to the back "karate chops"

Position and body use
- Stand behind your partner with one leg slightly in front of the other

Performing the technique
- Keeping your wrists relaxed, perform a chopping motion alternating hands and striking your partner's back with the side of the hand

- Think of the hand bouncing off your partner's back rather than into their body

- We suggest starting on the top edge of the right traps, moving medially toward the shoulder/neck junction, down the right erector spinae and then reversing this pattern on the left by going up the erector spinae to the shoulder and down the left trap

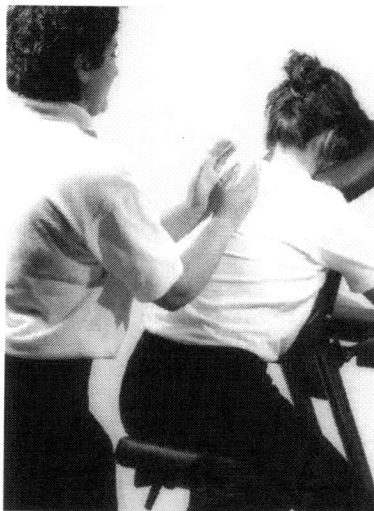

Other tips
- Because this is a more aggressive technique, perform it over fleshy areas like the shoulders, mid-back, and along the erector spinae muscles

- If you have troubles with the coordination of alternating hands, pretend that you are brushing dirt off your hands

- Keep your back aligned as you perform the technique to various places on the back or shoulders

- If you see your partner's body shaking or vibrating, you are hitting them too heavily

- To transition to the lower back, put one foot well behind the other and slowly lower onto one knee

21. Groove compression

Position and body use

- Stand behind and very slightly to one side of your partner

- Place the heel of the hand in the laminar groove

Performing the technique

- Let your weight fall into the heel of your hand then release the pressure

- Like all compression techniques, be sure that the force is directed at right angles to the back

- Lift the hand, move downward several inches and repeat

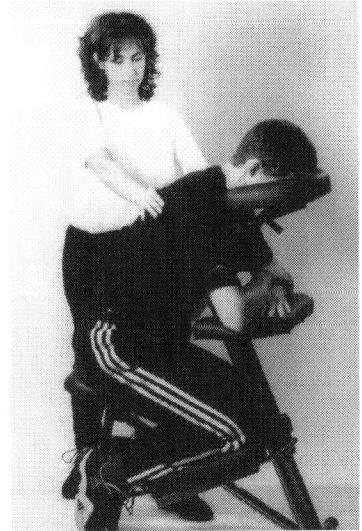

Other tips

- This technique is really designed to bow the erector spinae muscles to the side. Because there is not enough room in the groove for the heel of your hand, the erector spinae will naturally be compressed and will shift laterally from under your hand

- The upper back is usually too horizontal to let your weight fall forward effectively, so you'll likely need to use the strength in your arm muscles to do the compression for the first two or three compressions

22. Feathering

Position and body use

* Stand behind your partner

Performing the technique

* Using your whole hand, lightly stroke down the entire back several times in a slow soothing manner

* Be sure to include the neck and shoulders, and stroke all the way to the pelvis

Other tips

* You can use both hands simultaneously or alternate hands

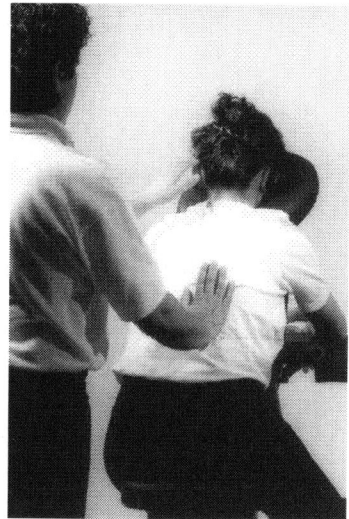

Accessory Techniques

We've called the following group of chair massage techniques *accessory techniques* simply because they are not part of the routine. These techniques can be used on their own or combined with the routine techniques. By doing so, you can create a customized massage for your client.

At the end of this list of techniques, we give you guidelines for tailoring a massage to meet your customer's needs.

Sanding

Position and body use

- Stand to the side of your partner

- Place your free hand gently on your partner's shoulder

- You can use various parts of your hand when doing this technique: the pads of the fingers, a relaxed fist, or the heel of your hand (illustrated in that order)

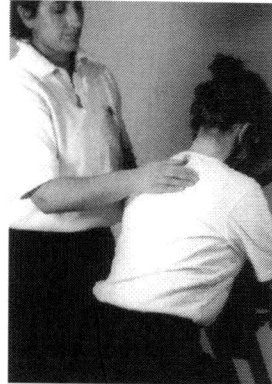

Performing the technique

- The technique is performed on the erector spinae between the spine and medial edge of the scapula on the opposite side of the back

- Slide your fingertips back and forth in a light, brisk way that resembles sanding wood with sandpaper.

- Continue slowly down the back

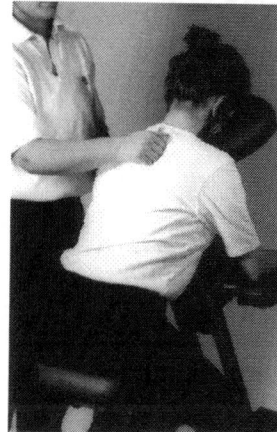

Other tips

- This technique is very superficial and your hand slides lightly over their clothing. Your partner shouldn't feel as if they are being pushed around in the chair

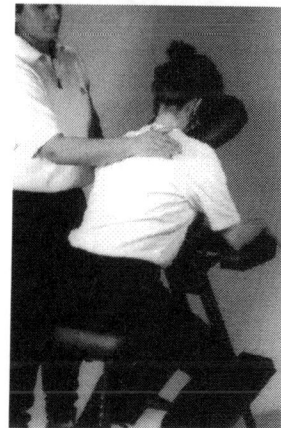

Spirals

Position and body use

- Stand to the side of your partner

- Place your hand gently in the middle of your partners back

- Use the full surface of your hand

Performing the technique

- Perform a circular motion with your hand starting in the middle of the back

- Make each subsequent circle increasingly larger until the circles cover the full width of the back

- Continue the circles making each one progressively smaller until your hand reaches the starting position

Other tips

- Like feathering, or sanding, this technique glides gently over the persons back

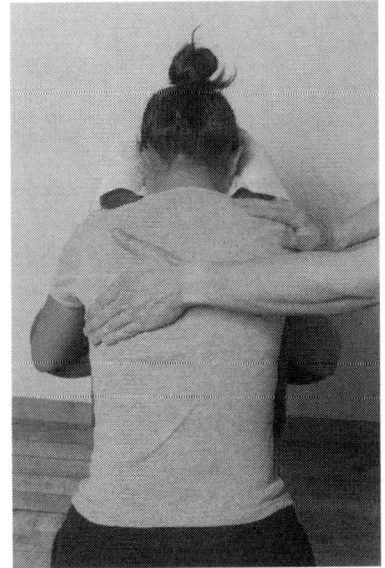

Back pressure points –Reinforced thumbs

Position and body use

- Reinforce the thumbs by placing one on top of the other

- Remember to keep your thumbs aligned in the direction of force by lining them up with your forearms.

Performing the technique

- Reinforce your thumbs and place them in the laminar groove

- Slowly and firmly press into the muscle, hold and then release

- Slide your thumbs down and perform a series of compressions down the back

- Go back to your starting position, move lateral a thumb width and repeat another row of compressions down the back

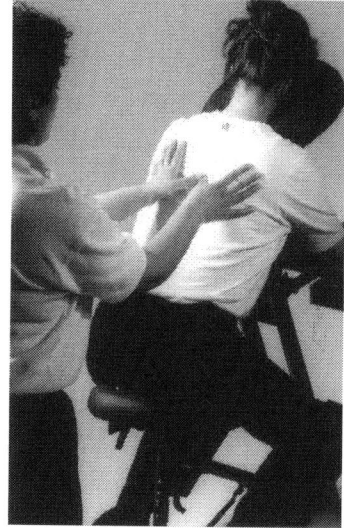

Other tips

- To keep your thumbs aligned, keep your palms off your partner's back. Use your index and middle finger to create a "tripod" with your thumb (as illustrated) or tuck your fingers in to make loose fists.

Back pressure points –Single thumb

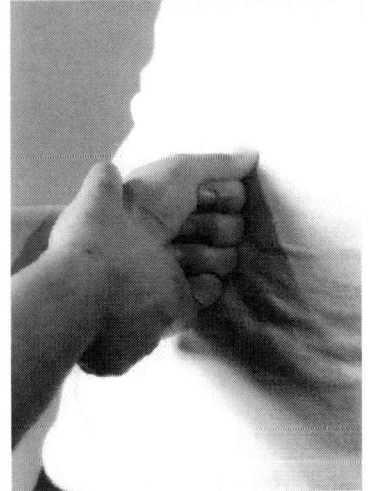

Position and body use

- Get into a lunge, slightly to the side of your partner

- If you are working on the right side, your right leg will be forward

- Make a loose fist with your left hand and place your thumb firmly against the side of your index finger

- Your thumb will extend slightly past the edge of the index finger to contact the back

- Wrap your right hand firmly around your left wrist for support

Performing the technique

- Keeping your thumb firmly on the side of your index finger and aligned with your forearm, let your weight all through your thumb

- Release the pressure slowly, lift the thumb and move to another point on the back

- Perform a series of compressions down the back

Other tips

- It's important to keep the thumb tightly against the index finger to prevent the thumb from hyperextending

- To maintain this position, you'll be using the tip of your thumb, so your nails must be short

- If your thumbs naturally hyperextend, then simply place your thumb between the index and middle finger to stabilize the distal joint (see photo)

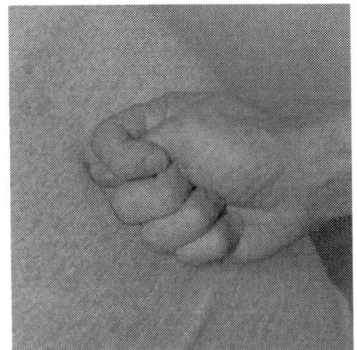

Back pressure points – Fists/Knuckles

Position and body use

- Get into a lunge, slightly to the side of your partner as you did with the single thumb compression above

- Make a fist with your left hand and place your fist on the back

- Keep your elbow directly behind your fist so that your wrist remains in a neutral alignment

- Wrap your right hand firmly around your left wrist for support

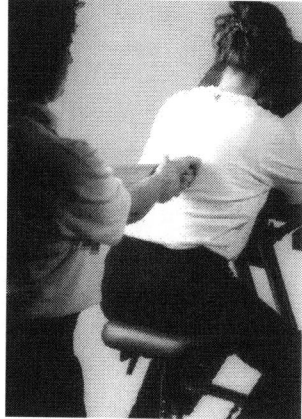

Performing the technique

- Let your weight all through your fist

- Release the pressure slowly, lift the fist and move to another point on the back

- Perform a series of compressions down the back

- Repeat on the other side

Other tips

- Avoid pressing on the spine or scapula

- This technique is relatively broad. For a more penetrating technique, use your knuckles.

When using your knuckles, move the elbow across the midline of the back so that the wrist remains in a neutral position

Back pressure points – Fist walking

Position and body use

- Stand behind your partner in a lunge position

- Place a fist on each side of the back

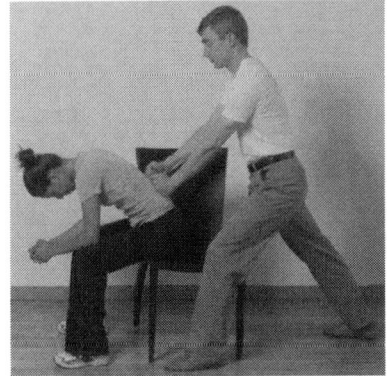

Performing the technique

- Let your weight fall through the fists

- Then lift one hand and place it several inches down the back

- Repeat with the other hand

- Continue this in a rhythmical way down the back in a way that resembles someone walking down their back

- Avoid pressing into the scapula or spinous processes

Other tips

- As with all compressions, always push into the body at right angles. This is particularly important in the upper back because it prevents your partner's neck from hyperextending

- Move up and down the back

- Isolate certain sections. For example, walk up and down the lumbar area only

- As you move into the low back, you'll find that you'll need to shift both the front and back leg back to provide space for your arms

Back Kneading - Thumb circles

Position and body use

- Stand behind your partner in a lunge position

- Place your thumbs about one inch lateral to the spinous processes

- Move the material and the skin toward the mid-line so that the thumbs are in the laminar groove directly besides the spinous processes

- It's vitally important that the thumbs stay aligned with the forearms throughout the movement

Performing the technique

- Press upwards and outwards in an arc across the erector spinae

- Release the pressure slightly as you complete the circle

- Be sure that the movement originates in the shoulders, not the thumbs

- Repeat this circular movement several times

- Lift the thumbs, move them down the back and repeat the sequence

Other tips

- The skin and the material should move with the thumbs throughout the movement. Do not glide over the material.

- To keep your thumbs aligned, keep your palms off your partner's back. Use your index and middle finger to create a "tripod" with your thumb (as illustrated for the *Back pressure points – Reinforced thumbs*) or tuck your fingers in to make loose fists.

Back Kneading – Bilateral elbow circles

Position and body use

- This is performed much like the *Thumb Circles*

- Stand behind your partner in a lunge position

- Place your elbows about one inch lateral to the spinous processes

- Rest your hands naturally on your shoulders

- Move the material and the skin toward the mid-line so that the elbows are in the laminar groove directly besides the spinous processes

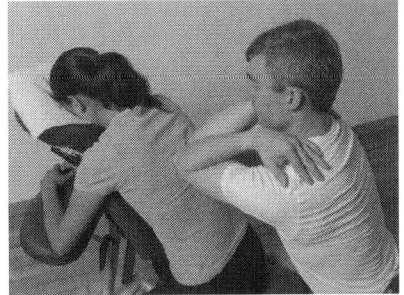

Performing the technique

- Press upwards and outwards in an arc across the erector spinae

- Release the pressure slightly as you complete the circle

- Repeat this circular movement several times

- Lift the elbows, move them down the back and repeat the sequence

Other tips

- The skin and the material should move with the elbows throughout the movement. Do not glide over the material.

- The biggest mistake made in performing the technique is to place the elbows too far lateral. When this is done, the kneading is done to the ribs rather than the erector spinae muscle

- Practitioners with broad shoulders or large breasts will not likely be able to get their elbows close enough together to perform this technique properly. They should perform the technique unilaterally (see below).

Back Kneading – Unilateral elbow circles

Position and body use

- Get into a lunge, slightly to the side of your partner

- If you are working on the right side, your right leg will be forward and you'll be using your left elbow

- Align yourself so that your shoulder is directly behind your elbow

- Place your elbow about one inch lateral to the spinous processes

- Move the material and the skin toward the mid-line so that the elbow is in the laminar groove directly besides the spinous processes

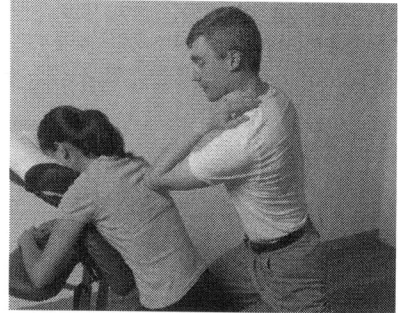

Performing the technique

- Press upwards and toward yourself in an arc across the erector spinae

- Release the pressure slightly as you complete the circle

- Repeat this circular movement several times

- Lift the elbow, move it down the back and repeat the sequence

Other tips

- The skin and the material should move with the elbows throughout the movement. Do not glide over the material.

- Again, be careful not to place the elbows too far lateral. Be sure the kneading is done over the erector spinae and not the ribs.

Fingertip frictions

Positioning and body use

- Get into a lunge, slightly to the side of your partner

- If you are working on the right side, your right leg will be forward and you'll be using your left fingers

- Align yourself so that your shoulder is directly behind your hand

- The fingertips contact the back while, your other hand forms a soft fist (placed on the back of the fingers) to reinforce your contact

Performing the technique

- Apply pressure as you move your fingers up and down without gliding or releasing the pressure

- Make the movement as big as you can without sliding over the shirt or skin

- It is very important to make the movement very even and rhythmical

- Repeat this up and down movement about 6 to 12 times in one spot

- Release the pressure, move down an inch and repeat the sequence

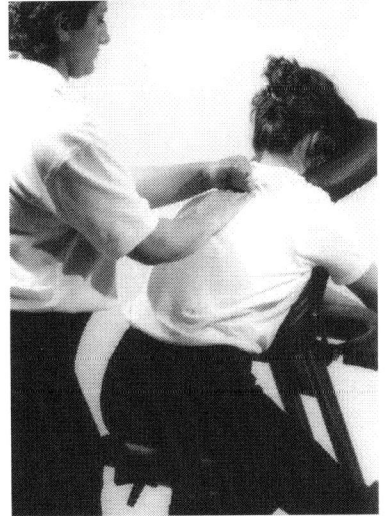

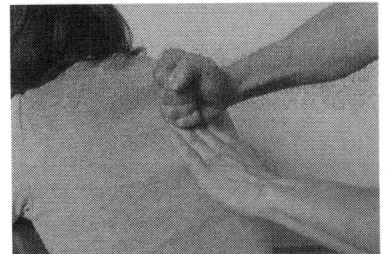

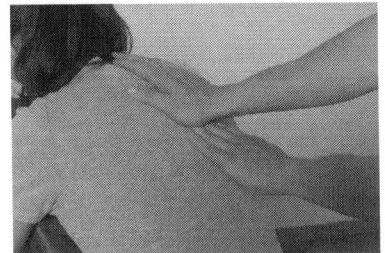

Other tips

- Like *Percussions*, the more the movement is repeated, the more relaxing it becomes

- You can also reinforce your fingertips with the fingertips of the other hand or with the heel of the hand

- Be sure to reinforce the distal phalanges. If you place your reinforcing fist or fingers too low, you'll force the finger joints into hyperextension

- Because there is no release phase in this technique, except for the short time to transition to the next point, only work one quadrant of the back at a time. Give your forearms a rest by using another technique before repeating the frictions on another quadrant.

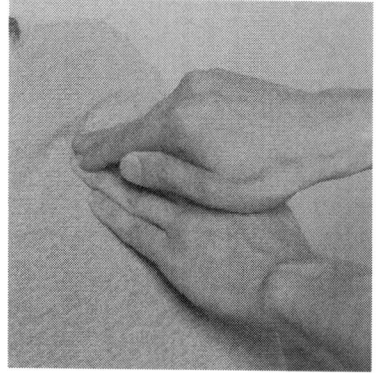

Fist/Knuckle frictions

- These are performed exactly in the same way as the fingertip frictions, except that the fist or the knuckles are used as a contact point.

- You can wrap your hand around the wrist of the working arm for support

- If using the knuckles, be sure to bring your elbow across the midline to help keep your wrist in a neutral alignment

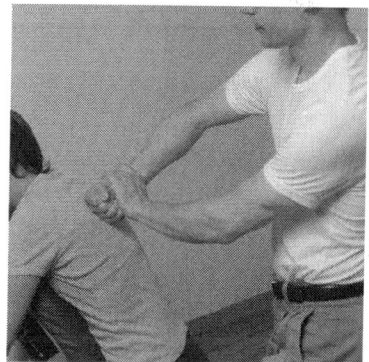

Three lines of elbow compression to the low back

Positioning and body use
- This technique is performed on the lower back.
- You should either be sitting or kneeling behind and slightly to the side your partner
- If you are slightly to the right of your partner, use your left elbow
- Start at the lower thoracic level and work downward

First line
- With your elbow in the laminar groove beside the spinous process, drop your hand across the mid-line and apply pressure in an outward direction against the medial border of the erector spinae muscles – pushing the erector spinae away from the spinous processes
- It is important to apply the pressure obliquely, pushing both forward and across. If you do not apply enough downward pressure, your elbow will roll over the erector spinae
- As you release the pressure slide down about an inch to the next point and repeat

Second line
- Position your elbow on the crest or ridge of the erector spinae muscle
- As with the elbow compression's to the shoulder, use your other hand in a v-shape to support the elbow and prevent it from falling off the crest of the erector spinae
- Push straight into the muscle with the elbow and slowly release
- Slide to the next point and repeat
- If you find that your elbow keeps rolling off the erector spinae, open the elbow, drop the hand laterally toward yourself slightly and press with the edge of the ulna

Third line
- Position your elbow along the lateral edge of the erector spinae
- Drop your hand slightly lateral and apply pressure against the outside edge of the erector spinae
- It is important to press at an oblique angle. If you push downward too much, you may press on the ribs. If you push across too much, you may roll over the erector spinae

QL Compressions

Position and body use

- Drop onto one knee – behind and slightly to the side of your partner

- Place your foot well away from the chair. To increase your force, you'll push this foot into the floor.

- Find the lateral edge of the Quadratus Lumborum (QL) between the ribs and pelvis. If you determine the width of the erector spinae at that level, simply place your elbow approximately twice that width from the spinous processes to locate the edge.

- Palpate firmly with your thumbs until you are better able to identify the edge with your elbow.

- Once you've located the edge with your thumbs, place your elbow on that point.

- Place your other hand on top of your fist as illustrated. Keep the elbow of that arm parallel to the floor.

- Your forearm should be at about a 45 degree angle to your partner's body.

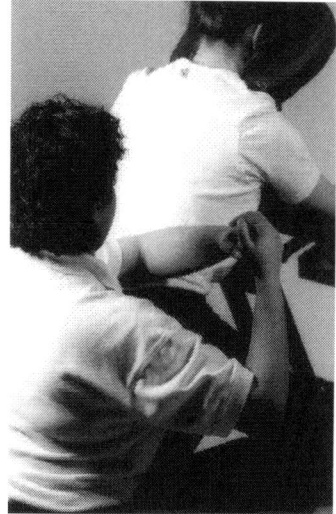

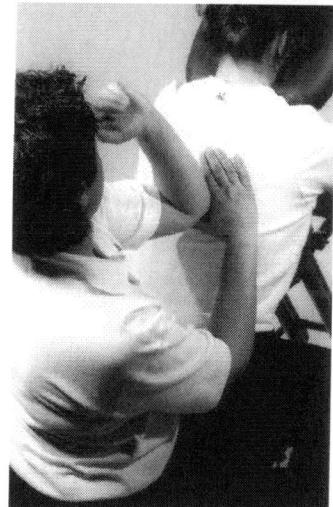

Performing the technique

- Press obliquely into the QL with your elbow.

- In this position, you'll be pushing into the belly of the muscle.

- To get the superior attachment of the QL at the ribs, keep your elbow in exactly the same position, but drop the hand downward so that the forearm is directed upwards slightly.

- To get the inferior attachment of the QL at the pelvis, keep your elbow in exactly the same position, but raise the hand upward so that the forearm is directed downward slightly.

Other tips

- To increase your force, press into your fist with your other hand and push your foot into the floor.

- Hold these compressions for some time – 10 to 20 seconds – to give the muscle time to relax under your elbow.

- There is very little space between the pelvis and the ribs, so you will not be able to move the elbow up or down along the edge of the muscle.

- The QL can often be very tender. The muscle attachments will be noticeably more tender than the belly of the muscle.

Fist compression to the shoulder

Position and body use

- Stand in front of your partner with your feet together

- Place your fists on the top edge of the trapezius muscle as close as possible to the neck

- Have your palms facing each other (i.e. thumbs are pointing posterior)

- Your elbows remain flexed so that the forearms are at right angles to the edge of the trapezius

Performing the technique

- Let your weight fall into your fists, release the pressure, move the fists outward slightly and repeat

- The compression is applied simultaneously to both shoulders

Other tips

- Be aware that as you approach the bony structures of the shoulder joint, you should lighten your pressure

- Push at right angles to the muscle (i.e. towards the opposite side of their seat) As an alternative, you can use the heel of your hands

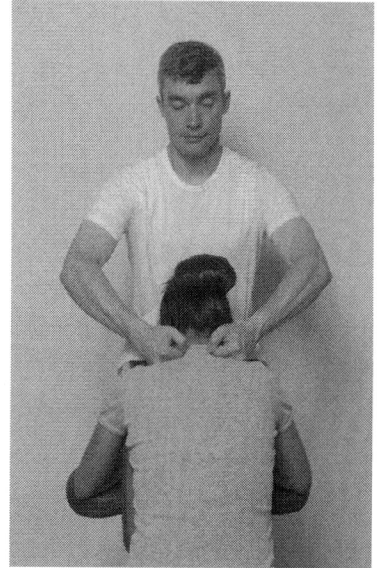

Pisiform circles to the neck shoulder junction

Position and body use

- Stand in front of your partner with your feet together

- Place your pisiforms on the levator scapula muscle as close as possible to the neck

- Your elbows remain flexed so that the forearms are at right angles to the edge of the trapezius

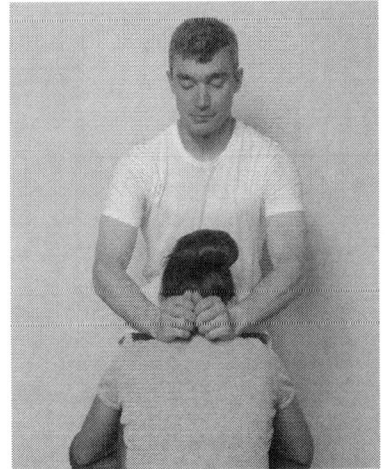

Performing the technique

- Let your weight fall into your pisiforms as they make and arc down the back and outward

- Only move as far as the skin and shirt allow

- Release the pressure slightly as you complete the circle to come back to your starting position

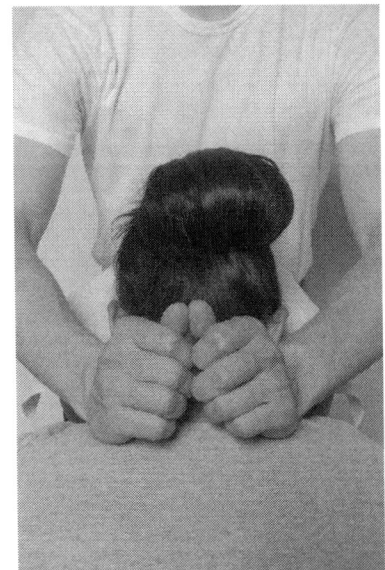

Other tips

- Be aware that as you approach the bony structures of the shoulder joint, you should lighten your pressure

- Don't slide over the shirt

Strumming the supraspinatus

Position and body use

- Stand to the side of your partner

- Place your thumb onto of the supraspinatus just medial to the acromioclavicular notch

- Reinforce the thumb with your other thumb or the fingers of the other hand (as illustrated)

Performing the technique

- Move the skin and shirt anterior so that the thumb is lying on the anterior edge of the supraspinatus. This gives you some slack in the skin and fabric

- Press firmly as you slide the thumb posterior

- If your thumb is positioned correctly, you'll feel yourself gently rolling or strumming over the supraspinatus

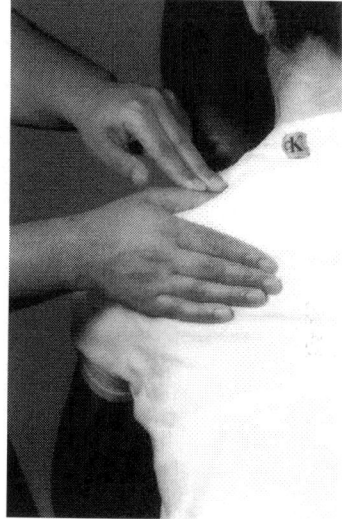

Other tips

- If the movement seems to abrupt, then simply direct the pressure medial as you strum back to perform more of a circular kneading action

Kneading the infraspinatus

Position and body use

- Kneel to one side of your partner

- Cup the front of the shoulder with the palm of your hand

- Place the pisiform of the working hand on the infraspinatus just below the spine of the scapula and lateral to the medial border

- Keep your elbows relatively high so that the force is generated from your chest muscles

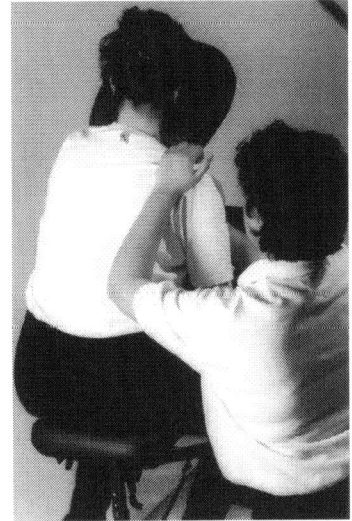

Performing the technique

- Perform a circular kneading action with the pisiform moving up and towards you

- Move your pisiform to another point in the infraspinous fossa and repeat

- Continue throughout the infraspinatus

Other tips

- Be sure to stay in the infraspinous fossa and avoid kneading bone. Often practitioners underestimate how much the shoulder blade drops forward when seated in the chair and will accidentally perform this technique over the medial edge of the scapula and even over the ribs

- Be sure to knead the tendon of the infraspinatus where it inserts into the humerus

Knuckle kneading to the neck – behind your partner

Position and body use

- Stand behind your partner

- Make a relaxed fist and place the second set of knuckles (the proximal interphalangeal joints) along the edge of the neck extensors

Performing the technique

- The movement of your hand and arm is a rolling/circular motion towards you. This is very similar to the C-Scoops that are part of the standard routine

- At each spot, the pressure is applied as you roll up the sides of the neck and towards yourself and then is released as the circular movement of your hands move away from you

- Lift your fists and move down to the next spot

- Start below the base of the skull and progress downwards towards the top of their shoulders

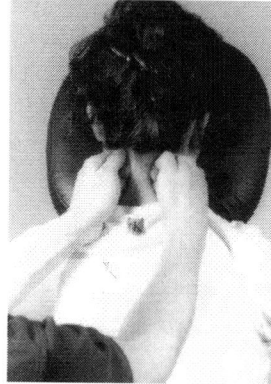

Other tips

- Avoid pushing the neck into extension. With this kneading action, the muscles are gently pulled away from the neck.

- You'll find that your fist is almost as wide as the neck is long and that you have very little distance to cover. So once you've gone as far along the neck extensors as you can go, continue the same kneading action across the top of the traps

- Although you are encouraged to use your core muscles as much as possible, you'll develop a smoother kneading action if you allow some of the circular movement to come from your wrists

Knuckle kneading to the neck – in front of your partner

Position and body use

- Stand in front of your partner with your feet together

- Make a relaxed fist and place the second set of knuckles (the proximal interphalangeal joints) along the edge of the neck extensors

- Because the knuckles lie at right angles to the edge of the extensors, you'll be isolating your contact to the side of the second or third finger.

- Start as far down the extensors as possible with the backs of your fingers resting on the top of the traps

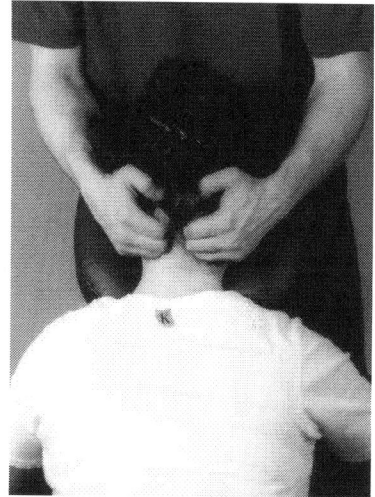

Performing the technique

- The movement of your hand and arm is exactly the same as if you were doing the technique behind your partner with a circular motion towards you. The difference is that the force phase of the movement is inferior and posterior instead of superior and posterior

- With each movement, catch the edge of the extensors with the side of the knuckle to gently pull the muscle away from the neck

- Lift your fists and move up to the next spot

- When your distal knuckles bump against the base of the skull, shift your contact point to the distal interphalangeal joints and continue kneading laterally across the base of the skull

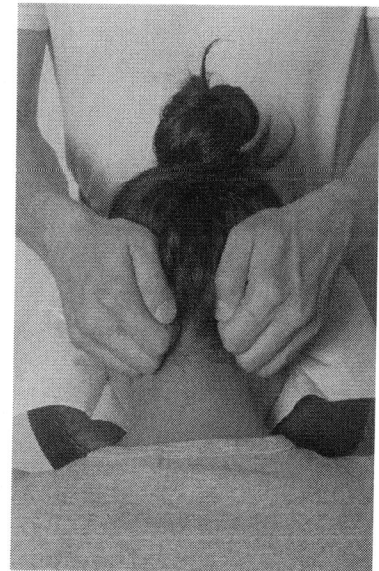

Other tips

- If you contact with all knuckles, you'll be pushing into the transverse processes, which will not be comfortable for your partner

- The kneading across the base of the skull resembles the thumb kneading. With each movement the neck is gently pulled into flexion

- Keep your wrists relaxed. Allow some of the circular movement to come from your wrists

Pinching to the neck extensors

Position and body use

- Stand on to the side of your partner and place your hand on their opposite trapezius

- Start by facing the same direction as your partner and standing a little behind them

- To maintain the proper alignment of your hand as you do this series of squeezes up the neck, you'll need to gradually move anterior until you are standing beside the arm rest

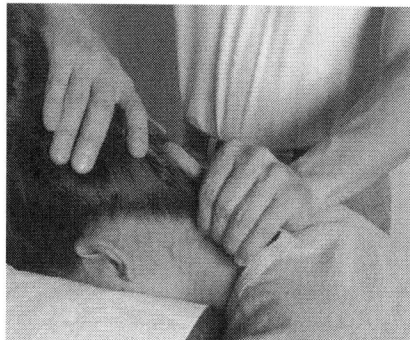

Performing the technique

- Start by draping your hand over the trapezius muscle as if you are doing a one-handed *Trap Squeeze*

- Squeeze and release between the heel of the hand and the fingertips

- Move the hand medial and repeat

- Continue moving up the extensors. As you move from the traps to the neck extensors as a whole, place the heel of your thumb on the top of the spinous processes with the thumb pointing upwards and place the fingertips of your first two or three fingers on the front edge of the neck extensor muscles

- Squeeze so that you catch the medial and lateral edges of the extensors and release

Other tips

- This technique is performed to the opposite side of the neck

- Gently press the heel of the thumb into the spinous processes as you begin the squeeze so that the metacarpal of your thumb scoops under and catches the medial edge of the extensors. If you let the heel of the thumb slide over the top of the muscle, you'll end up pinching skin rather than squeezing the muscle

- As you go up the neck, be sure to grab all the extensors and not just the edge of the traps

Fingertip walking base of skull – short strokes

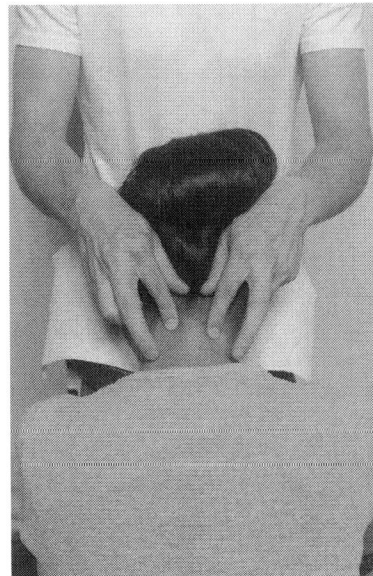

Position and body use
- Stand in front of your partner
- Place the heels of the hands on the base of the skull and let your fingers rest down the neck. The heels of your hands remain in the same position on the skull throughout the movement

Performing the technique
- Press one index finger firmly into the neck directly beside the spinous processes and maintain the pressure as you slowly slide the finger to the base of the skull
- As that index finger approaches the base of the skull, start the same movement with the other index finger
- Continue alternating the fingers this way for several repetitions
- Because the heels of the hand remain on the base of the skull, these movements are quite short
- Then switch to the middle finger and perform the same movement by alternating the middle fingers. You are now a finger width away from the spinous processes. Continue for several repetitions and then switch to the ring finger

Other tips
- Slide slowly so that you do not burn the skin. Stop when you bump up against the base of the skull. Don't slide any further or you'll pull their hair
- By using each of these three fingers, you are covering the entire width of the neck extensors
- Don't try to bend over your partner's head to watch your fingers. Stand in a relaxed, upright position
- To finish off this technique, slide all fingers up the neck together until they come up against the base of the skull, then let your weight gently fall back to place a traction the skull and provide a gentle stretch to the neck extensors

Fingertip walking base of skull – long strokes

Position and body use

- Stand in front of your partner

- Place the pad of the middle fingers on the nail of the index fingers to reinforce the fingers

- Place the index fingers beside the spinous processes at the C7 level

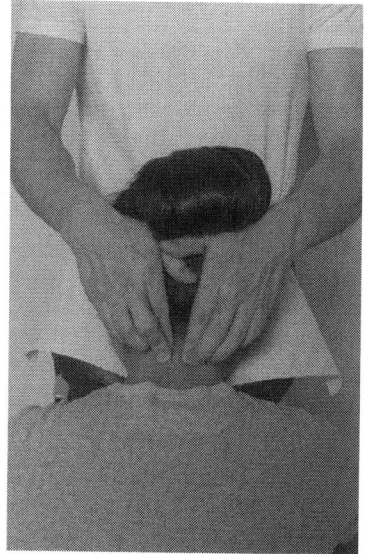

Performing the technique

- Press the index fingers firmly into the neck directly beside the spinous processes and maintain the pressure as you slowly slide the fingers to the base of the skull

- When you reach the base of the skull, pause momentarily maintaining some slight traction to the skull

- Slowly release both fingers, return to the starting position and move them outward a finger width

- Press into the neck as you slide the fingers upward

- Repeat this sequence several times moving a little more lateral with each subsequent movement

Other tips

- Slide slowly to avoid burning the skin

- Unlike the *short strokes* that focus on the suboccipital area only, these *long strokes* move up the entire length of the neck

- Stay on top of the extensor muscles. If you move too far lateral, you'll be pushing against the sides of the vertebra

Arm jiggle

- Have your partners arm by their side

- Curve your relaxed hand around your partner's upper arm

- Use your whole hand, not just the fingertips, to jiggle the arm muscles

- Gently jiggle the arm by flopping your hand in and out, keeping your hand in contact with the arm at all times

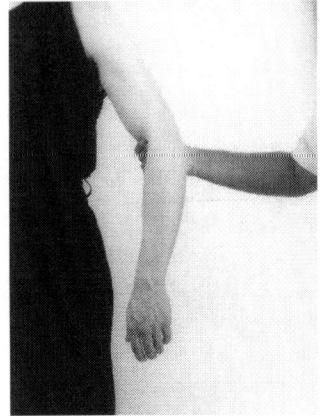

Bread roll

- Place your partner's arm between your two flat hands

- Roll the arm between your hands like rolling out bread dough into breadsticks

- Slowly roll from the armpit down to the wrist

- Repeat two to three times

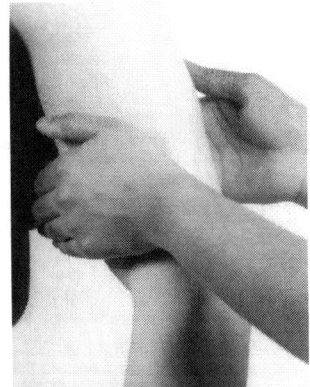

Spreading the palm

- Turn the palm of the hand to face you

- Put your fingers under your partner's hand and rest the heels of your thumbs on the palm, directly over the carpal bones

- Push the heels of your thumbs downward as the fingers push upward in a way that resembles breaking a popsicle in half

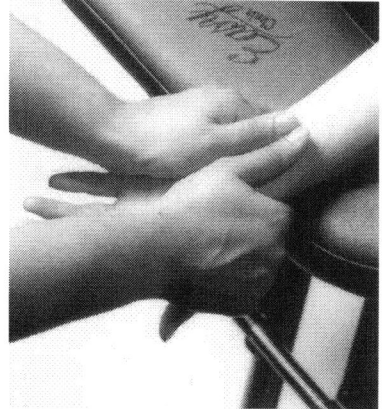

Spreading the palm II

- With your partners palm facing away from you, place your fingers on the palm of the hand and rest the heels of your thumbs on top of the hand

- Spread the palmar surface of the hand by sliding your fingers outwards in a way that resembles breaking a popsicle in a reverse direction

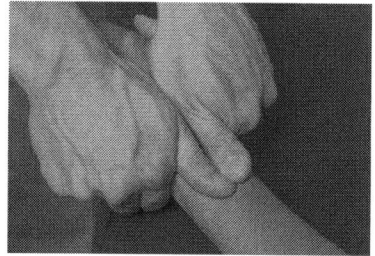

Thumb compression to palm (fast and alternating)

- Place the flats of your fingers under the dorsal surface of the hand and place the pads of your thumbs on the palm

- Perform a walking action with your thumbs on the palm of the hand

- Move the thumbs relatively fast and cover the entire palm

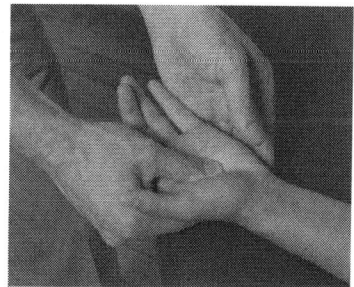

Finger squeezes

- Place your partner's hand loosely in your hand

- Grasp the base of one of your partner's finger and gently squeeze each small segment between the joints top to bottom, moving out toward the tip of the finger

- Repeat to each finger

- Then repeat squeezing side to side

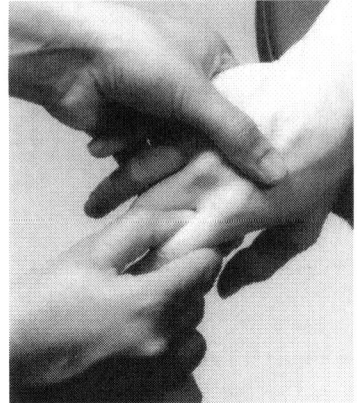

Feather stroke to the arm

- Gently stroke down the entire arm as is done with the feather stroke technique to the back

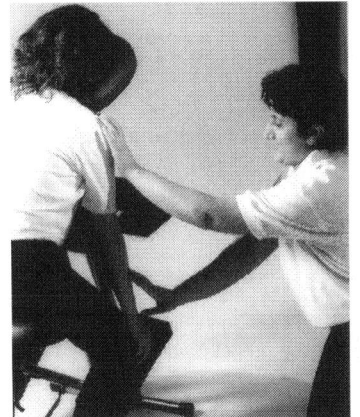

Techniques for the Upright Seated Position

In some cases, your customer may not be able to sit in the massage chair. For example, a senior with limited mobility or some who is in a wheel chair. Other times, a customer may simply not want to sit in the chair. Some customers, for example, may not want to leave their desks and some women may be afraid of messing up their makeup.

In these cases you will have to adapt your techniques so that you can massage the person sitting upright without the support of the massage chair. In this section you'll find a number of techniques that can be used for this purpose. In addition, your instructors will show you how to adapt many of the techniques that you've already learned.

Because the chair is not supporting the customer's body, you have to provide support. You are often unable to utilize your body weight in the same way with the person in the chair. For those reasons, this type of massage much more challenging and much more physical.

When you are working on the back, you will often have to support your customer across the front of the chest. Cup your hand loosely over the opposite shoulder. Be careful not to clutch that shoulder with your fingers. Keep your body low so that the forearm does not come up across the neck and choke your partner.

When you are working on the neck, put one hand on the forehead and get your customer to drop the head forward into your hand. Keep your elbow tucked into your side to prevent your support arm from becoming fatigued. Pay attention to the support hand so that your fingers are not dropping into their eyes or that your hand is not stretching the skin on the forehead upward.

Forearm compressions to traps

Position and body use

- Have your partner sit upright in the chair

- Stand behind your partner with your feet together to keep your center of gravity high

Performing the technique

- Rest your forearms on top of your partner's shoulders beside the neck contacting as close to your elbow as possible

- Slowly let your weight fall straight down onto your partner's shoulders

- Release slowly, shift lateral and repeat

Other tips

- As you move outward along the shoulders be sure to pronate the forearms. This allows the fleshy part of the forearm to make contact and prevents your ulna from pressing into the bone at the outer edge of the shoulder

Variations

You can do the compressions on just one side at a time (unilateral). If you are doing a unilateral compression, then stand to one side of your partner and use the forearm closest to your partners back. Be sure to direct your pressure toward the opposite side of the pelvis.

You can also do the unilateral compressions with your partner leaning forward in the chair. In this case, stand in a lunge facing and slightly to the side of your partner. Use the forearm that is closest to your partner.

Compressions to the inside edge of the shoulder blade

- Brace the front of your partners shoulders

- Locate the top corner of the opposite shoulder blade and place the heel of your hand just below this point and compress against the medial edge of the shoulder blade

- Slide your hand down slightly and repeat the sequence until you have reached the bottom corner of the shoulder blade

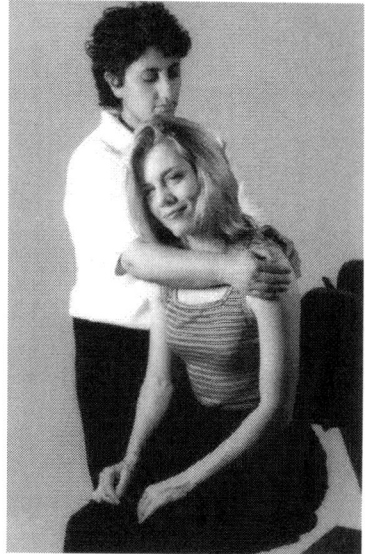

The claw

- You can stand to one side of your partner or behind your partner

- Place all your fingertips on your partner's skull

- Make gentle, slow circles, moving the skin of the scalp over the underlying bone.

Note: Vary your contact point, don't dig your fingernails into the scalp. Apply enough pressure so that you don't slide over the hair.

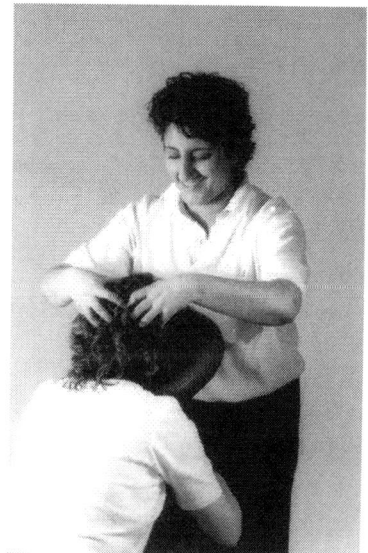

Hair pulling

- Be gentle with this technique

- Grab large clumps of hair in a loose fist

- Pull the hair away from the skull.

- Release and repeat.

Supporting the Head

For these next techniques you will need to support your partner's head. Have them lean their head back against you. Make sure that your partner doesn't hyperextend their neck in doing so. You will have a tendency to do this so that you can see what your hands are doing. You may want to take a pillow or the chest pad from the chair and place it between your body and your partner's head.

Kneading to the temples

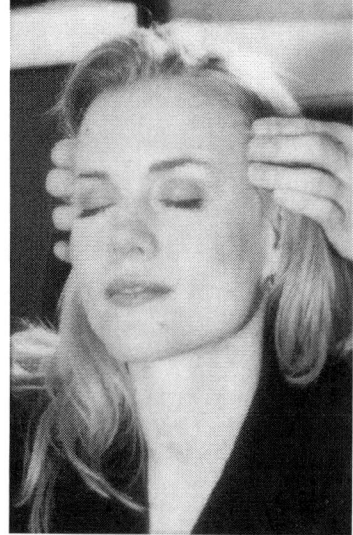

- Start with your fingertips approximately one inch lateral to the outer corner of the eye

- Using the fat pads of your fingertips knead the temples

- Apply pressure as you perform the circular movements moving the skin over the underlying bone

- Repeat the circular movement three to four times before moving to the next position

- Perform this technique over the temporalis muscle

Note: you can continue the circular kneading across the forehead

Forehead spread

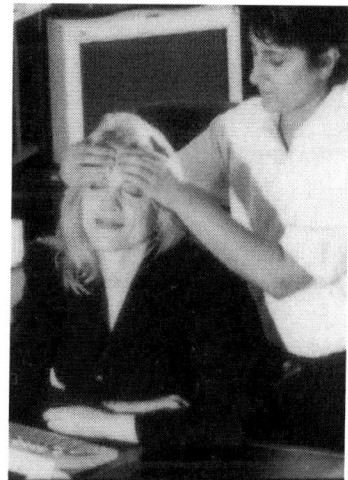

- Locate the mid-line of the forehead

- Align your fingertips of your right and left hand at the mid-line

- Slide your fingertips will some pressure laterally out to the temples

- Repeat two or three times

Finger kneading to the jaw

- Place the flat pads of your fingertips one-inch in front of the ear and below the zygomatic arch on either side of the face.

- Perform several small circular movement with the fingertips on the jaw

- Repeat the circular kneading bilaterally over the masseter muscle

Stripping to the jaw

- Place the heels of the thumbs below the zygomatic arch as above

- Apply a gentle pressure as you slide the heels of the thumbs straight down the sides of the jaw

- Do not slide forward toward the chin

- Repeat two to three times keeping the pressure consistent

Tapping to the head

- Finish the head by gently tapping your fingertips over the skull, forehead, cheeks and jaw

Lower body techniques

For the lower body techniques, you will have to get onto the floor. There are several positions that you can take depending on what technique you are performing and what is most comfortable for you. You may kneel on one knee, kneel sitting on your feet or with your buttocks partly raised off your feet, sit with your legs crossed or sit with one or both legs extended in front of you. The pictures that accompany the following descriptions do not show all the possible variations for body position. Experiment and find out what works best for you.

Most of the techniques described below are done with the person's leg off the shin rest. The leg is pulled slightly away from the chair and the person's foot is placed flat on the ground. Most of these techniques can be adapted so that they can be done with the person's leg on the shin rest. But by removing the leg from the support, you will have better access and will be able to use your body more effectively.

Although some of these techniques look invasive, they actually feel quite safe for the individual in the chair. Start the techniques as proximal as you can on the thigh being careful when working the medial thigh.

Cupped hand squeeze to the quads

- Kneel to the side of you partner at right angles to the thigh

- Place cupped hands side by side over the top of the thigh

- Squeeze the quadriceps muscle between the flats of your fingers and the heel of your hand

- Push downwards as you squeeze to get more muscle into your hand and to avoid pinching your partner

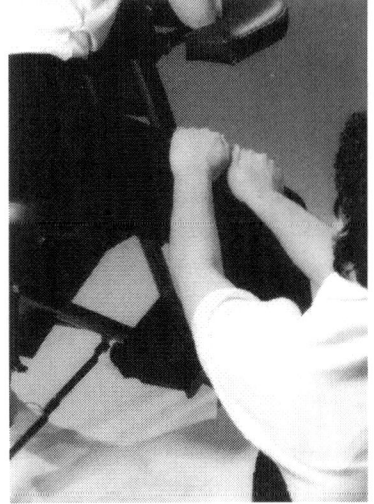

- ■

Interlaced squeeze to the quads

- Position your body in front of your partner's knee so that your body is in alignment with their thigh

- Interlace your fingers

- Place the heels of the hands on each edge of the quadriceps and squeeze the muscle between the heel of your hands

- Keep your elbows up as much as possible so that the force comes from your chest. However, you may have to drop the inside arm because of limited space

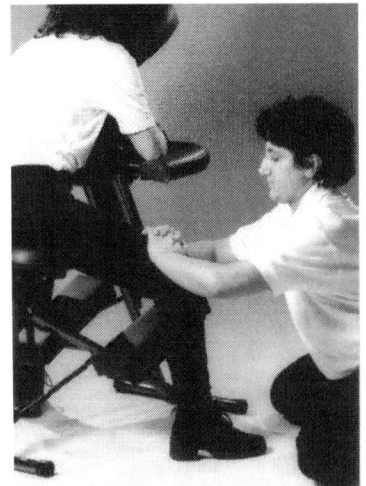

Open arm compression to thigh

- Position yourself in front of your partner's knee

- Open up the interlaced fingers bringing the heels of your hand to the medial and lateral thigh

- The heels of the hands are directly opposite to each other on the IT band and the adductor muscles

- Compress the medial and lateral thigh with the heel of your hands by pushing the hands toward one another

- Keep the elbows up as much as possible

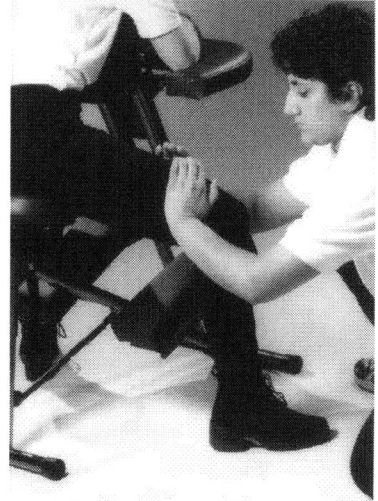

Adductor squeeze

- Kneel to the side of you partner at right angles to the thigh

- Place one hand flat like a ledge on the inside of the thigh, under the adductors; place it just medial to the hamstrings

- Put the heel of the other hand just medial to the edge of the quadriceps

- Use this hand to compress the adductors against the heel of your lower hand

- Repeat the compression from the top of the leg down towards the knee

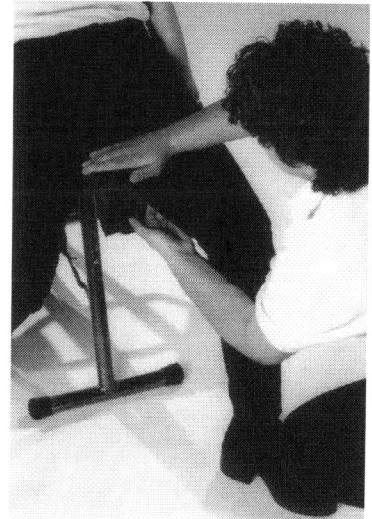

IT Band compression – fist

- Make a fist

- Using the back of the fist, push firmly into the IT band along the lateral thigh

- Stabilize the leg by placing the palm of your free hand flat on the medial knee

- Do a series of compressions along the lateral thigh

- You can position yourself at right angles to the thigh or in front of the knee

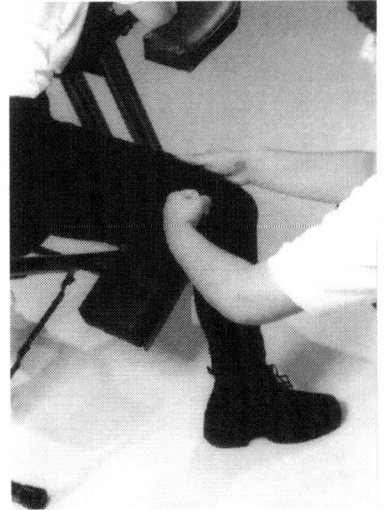

IT Band compression -- heel of hand

- Using the heel of your hand, push firmly into the IT band along the lateral thigh

- Stabilize the leg by placing the palm of your free hand flat on the medial knee

- Do a series of compressions along the lateral thigh

- You can position yourself at right angles to the thigh or in front of the knee

- Note that this is a smaller contact point and will feel more penetrating than the fist compressions

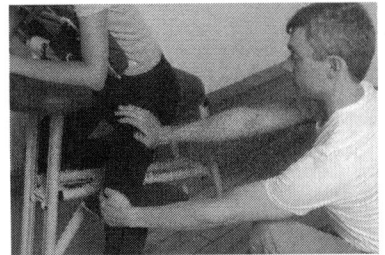

Fist compression to the gluteus muscles - unilateral

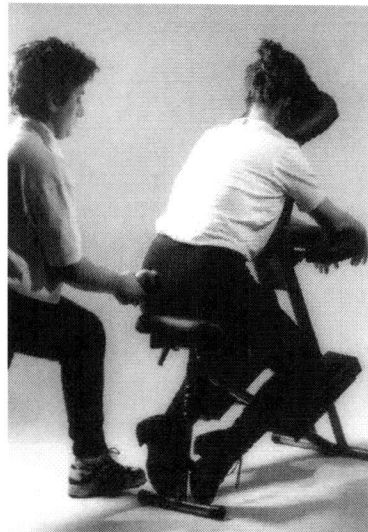

- Position yourself so that you are kneeling beside and slightly behind your partner (kneeling on one knee will work best for this particular technique)

- Make a fist with one hand and wrap your other hand around your wrist for support

- Place your fist in the gluteus muscles and let your weight fall forward through the arm

- Do a series of compressions throughout the gluteus

- Make sure you are compressing muscle by staying below the level of the iliac crest (hipbones)

- For a more penetrating compression let the weight fall through your knuckles specifically instead of the backs of the fingers

- The lateral gluteus muscles (medius and minimus) are often quite tender

Fist compression to the gluteus muscles – bilateral

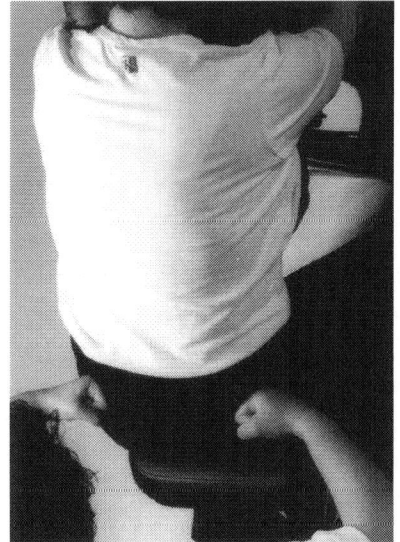

- Position yourself directly behind your partner

- Place one fist on each side of the buttocks

- Keep your elbows high so that the force comes from your chest

- Push your fists towards each other

- Do a series of compressions throughout the gluteus

- Make sure you are compressing muscle by staying below the level of the iliac crest (hipbones)

- For a more penetrating compression let the weight fall through your knuckles specifically instead of the backs of the fingers

- The lateral gluteus muscles (medius and minimus) are often quite tender

Cupped hand squeeze to the hamstrings

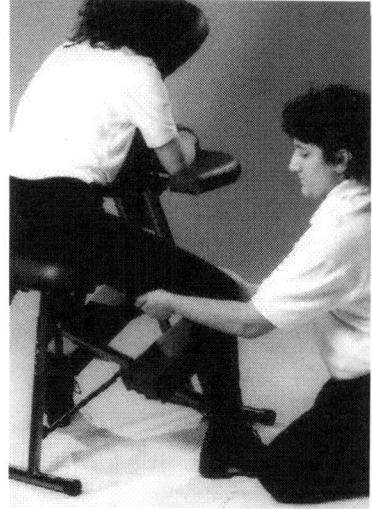

- Kneel to the side of you partner at right angles to the thigh

- Place one hand on top of the knee for support

- Cup the other hand and place it under the thigh so that your fingers and heel of hand are on the edges of the hamstring muscles

- Push upwards to push the muscle into your hand as you squeeze between your fingers and the heel of your hand

- Do a series of squeezes moving up or down the thigh

Hamstring shake

- Cup the hamstring in one hand

- Gently shake from side to side with a loose, easy shake

Interlaced squeeze to the hamstrings

- Position yourself in front of your partner's knee

- Interlace your fingers under your partner's thigh

- Place the heels of the hands on each side of the hamstring muscles

- Squeeze the hamstrings between the heel of the hands

- Do a series of squeezes moving up or down the thigh

Interlaced squeeze to calves

- Position yourself in front of your partner's knee

- Interlace your fingers behind your partner's calf

- Place the heels of the hands on each side of the calf muscle

- Squeeze the calf between the heel of the hands

- Do a series of squeezes starting the squeezes below the knee and finishing at the Achilles tendon

- The calf muscle narrows as it reaches the heel. Make sure that the heels of your hands remain on the edges of the muscle so that you don't end up squeezing the bone

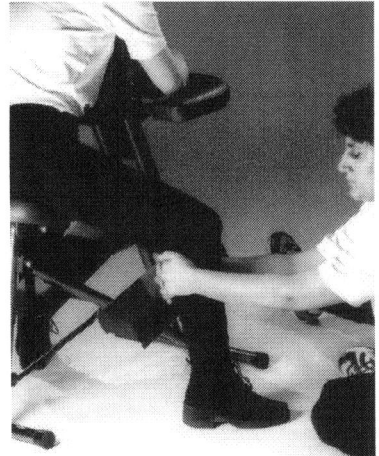

Medial calf squeeze

- Position yourself in front of your partner's knee
- Cup one hand over the medial calf muscle placing the fingertips in the middle of the calf and the heel of the hand on the medial edge
- Squeeze between the fingers and the heel of the hand
- Do a series of squeezes moving up or down the calf
- The calf muscle narrows towards the ankle so be sure that your contact points remain on the edges of the muscle

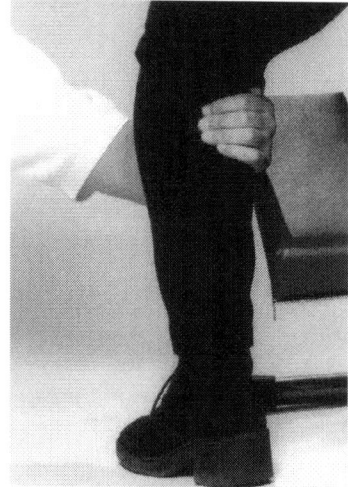

Lateral calf squeeze

- Position yourself in front of your partner's knee
- Cup one hand over the lateral calf muscle placing the fingertips in the middle of the calf and the heel of the hand on the medial edge
- Squeeze between the fingers and the heel of the hand
- Do a series of squeezes moving up or down the calf
- Note that the lateral aspect of the calf is much smaller than the medial

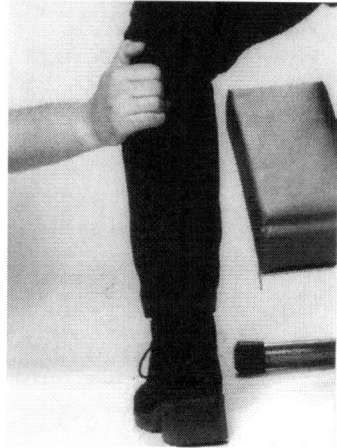

Alternating calf squeezes

- Cup your hands over medial and lateral calf muscles as above
- Do alternate squeezes up or down the lower leg

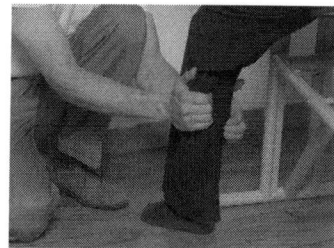

Fingertip compressions to calf

- Place your fingertips on the midline of the calf muscles so that the nails of one hand are against the nails of the other

- Starting just below the knee, gently compress the muscle with the fingertips by letting your weight fall backwards

- Move down one inch and repeat the compression until you reach the Achilles tendon

- As an alternative, keep the leg on the shin rest and do the compressions with reinforced thumbs

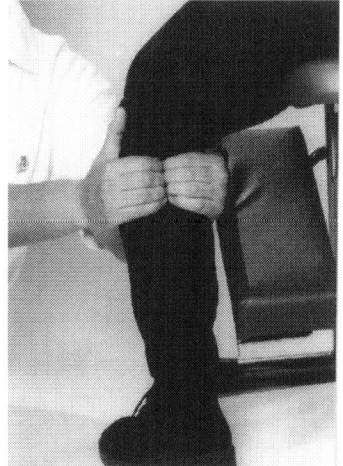

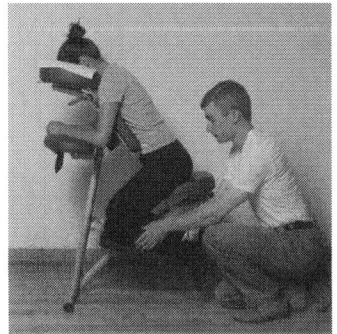

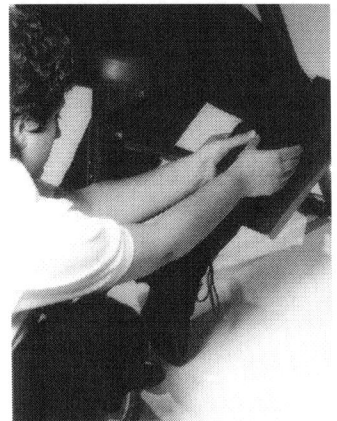

Compartment compressions

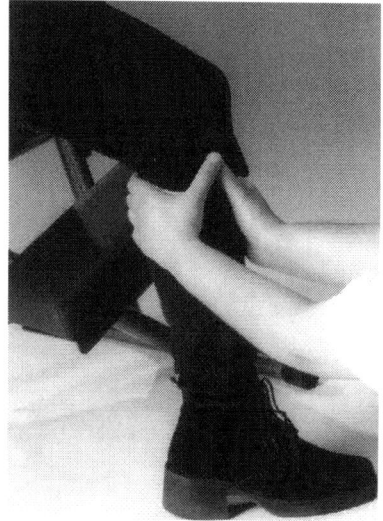

- These thumb compressions will be done in the anterior and lateral "compartments" of the lower leg

- Place your thumbs on the muscle below the knee and just lateral to the shin bone (tibia)

- Do a series of compressions in a line downward using reinforced thumbs

- Once you've reached the inferior end of the compartment, bring your thumbs one inch lateral to the starting position and repeat a series of compressions moving down the lower leg

- You will perform several lines of compressions like this, moving laterally with each column until you are on the most lateral aspect of the lower leg

Bread roll to leg

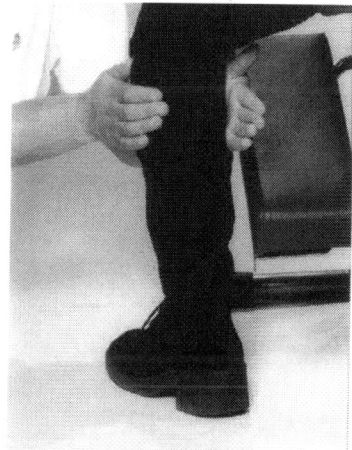

- Place the flats of the hands on each side of the calf

- Roll the leg between your open palms, like a breadstick.

Feathering to leg

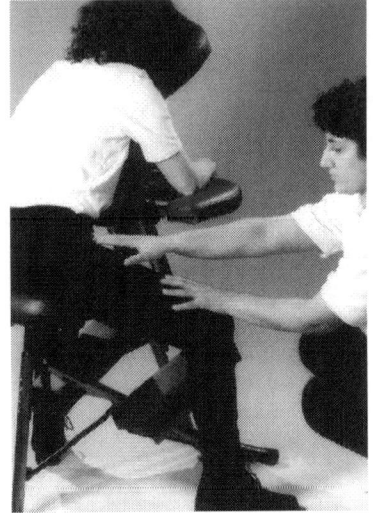

- Using the broad surface of the hand stroke down the leg

- You can do the feathering to the thigh, to the lower leg or the entire leg

- Avoid being too superficial with your touch because many people are ticklish on their legs

- You can use both hands simultaneously or alternate the hand contact

Compression to sole of foot

Thumb compressions

- Place the leg on the shin rest

- Place the flats of your fingers on the top (dorsal surface) of the foot

- Reinforce your thumbs and compress into the bottom (plantar surface) of the foot

- Do a series of compressions through the fleshy areas of the foot and particular the arch

- Move slowly and press firmly to avoid tickling your partner's feet

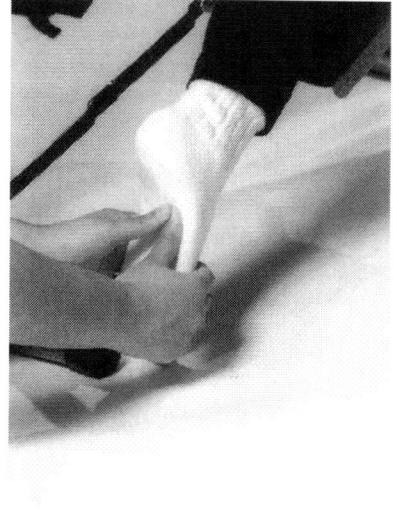

Fist compressions

- Place the leg on the shin rest

- Use one hand to support the top of the foot

- Make a fist with the other hand and press firmly into the sole of the foot

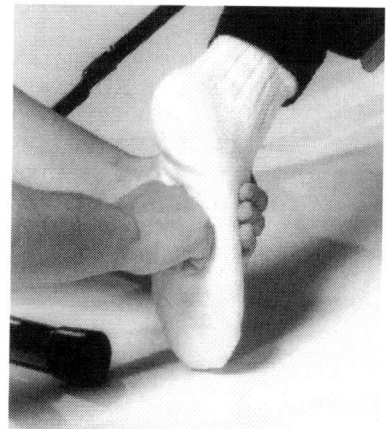

Fingertip compressions

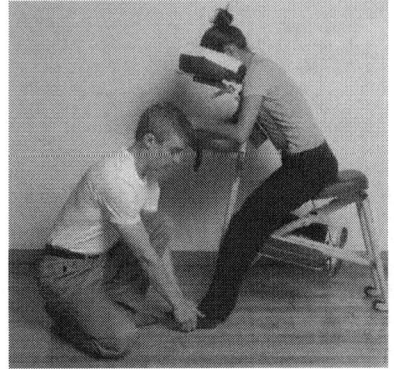

- Place the foot flat on the ground

- Extend the knee slightly so that you can dorsiflex the ankle to get your hands under the foot

- Place the heels of your hands on top of the foot and wrap your fingers underneath

- Press up into the sole of the foot with your fingertips

- Press firmly and move slowly around the sole of the foot

- Use more specific pressure by letting the weight fall through your knuckles rather than the backs of the fingers

- You can press with both sets of fingertips at the same time or alternate hands

Shaking to metatarsals

- Grasp the heads of two adjacent metatarsals between the thumb and index fingers

- Be sure to grab just proximal to the knuckle

- Push one metatarsal away as you pull the other toward you and reverse

- Do this at a quick rate so that you are shaking the metatarsals back and forth

- Shift each hand over to the next metatarsals and repeat across the foot

- This is similar to the Metacarpal Shake done to the hand

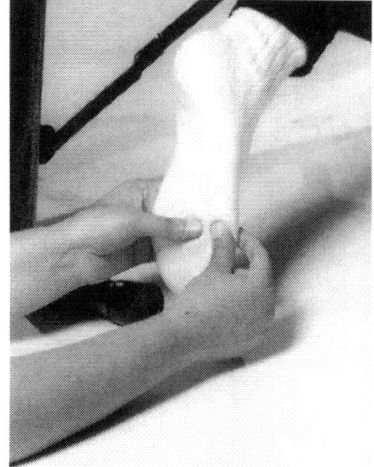

Squeezes to toes

- Support the foot with one hand

- Grasp a toe between the thumb and the side of the index finger over the proximal phalange

- Squeeze gently

- Do several squeezes to the toe moving distally with each squeeze

- Repeat to each toe

- You can also squeeze the sides of the toes in the same way although this is difficult to do unless your partner has bare feet

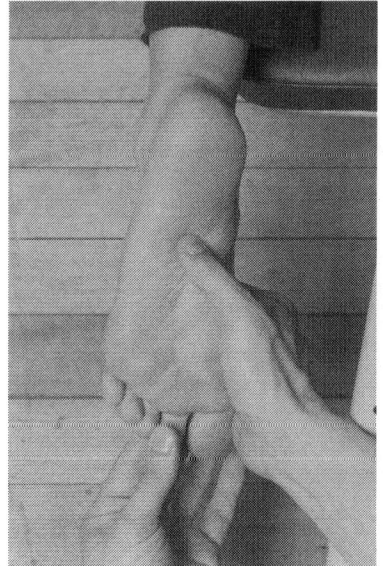

Traction to toes

- Grasp the base of one of your partner's toes between your thumb and index finger

- Keep the thumb in line with the toe and maintain a broad contact

- Firmly pull on the toe

- Repeat to all toes

- As a variation, as you traction the toe, roll the toe back and forth between the finger and thumb

Foot squeezes

- Wrap both hands around the foot

- Squeeze the foot using the broad surfaces of the fingers and hands

- This can be done with the leg on the shin rest or with the foot flat on the floor

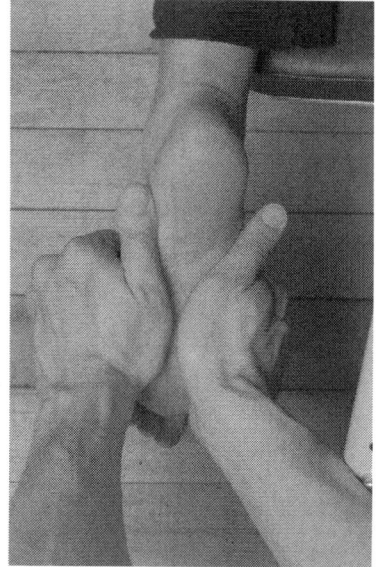

Bread roll to foot

- With leg on shin rest, place the flats of the hands on each side of the foot

- Quickly roll the foot back and forth between the hands

- Be careful not to pull the leg off the shin rest

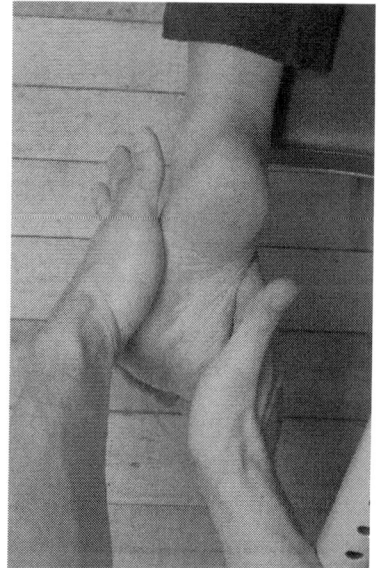

Stretches

Here are a number of stretches that you can use to help stretch out tight muscles in the neck and chest. These muscles in particular have a tendency to get tight in people who are sedentary.

These stretches are potentially the most "dangerous" of all the techniques that you will learn in the course. You use the bones as levers and can generate a great deal of force with a minimal amount of effort. Make sure that the person is comfortable throughout these stretches. Be sure that they know that they should not feel pain during these stretches. The stretch sensation should be pleasant and comfortable. Be on the lookout for non-verbal cues that indicate that your client may be uncomfortable with the stretch, such as flinching, shifting positions and resisting the movement.

With all stretches, bring the arm or limb through the movement described and elicit feedback as you reach the end of the movement. Don't ask: "Is this OK?" As we know, customers will be hesitant to give you accurate feedback if they feel that they are criticizing you. Instead ask, "Are you feeling a comfortable stretch? or do we need to stretch a little further?"

When you've reached the point where they are feeling a comfortable stretch, hold that position for five to ten seconds. Do not force the movement. Do not bounce. Doing so is not only potentially dangerous, but will cause the muscle to tighten.

Assist their head to an upright position or assist them in bringing their arm back to their side. Why? Because after the muscle has been stretched, it will be weak momentarily and you will want to be sure that they have as much support as they need as they come back to a neutral position. This will prevent them from straining their muscles.

Caution: Absolutely do not do the pectoralis stretch on anyone with a previous shoulder dislocation. Always ask your client before you do the stretch whether or not they have ever dislocated their shoulder.

Upper Trap Stretch

- Stand behind your partner

- Assist your partner into an upright seated position

- With your elbow bent, rest your forearm on top of your partner's left shoulder (a few inches medial to the bony area) - this is to prevent this side from raising while you perform the stretch to the opposite side

- Tell your partner where they should be feeling the stretch and ask them to tell you as soon as they start to feel a slight or gentle stretch

- Instruct your partner to drop their ear to their right shoulder (opposite to the side you are stabilizing the shoulder with your forearm)

- Be sure your partner's neck is straight and their chin is tucked in

- If they do not indicate that they are feeling a stretch, ask them if they are feeling anything

- If your partner is not feeling a stretch, tell your partner that you are going to apply a gentle pressure to the side of their head to assist in the stretch

- Do this very slowly and clearly ask your partner to tell you when they are feeling the stretch. Do not proceed with this step unless your partner has told you that they are not feeling a stretch from their own efforts

- Hold for 5 seconds, encouraging your partner to breath slowly and deeply

- While continuing to stabilize the shoulder, use the other forearm to support the side of your partner's head and gently assist their head into an upright position

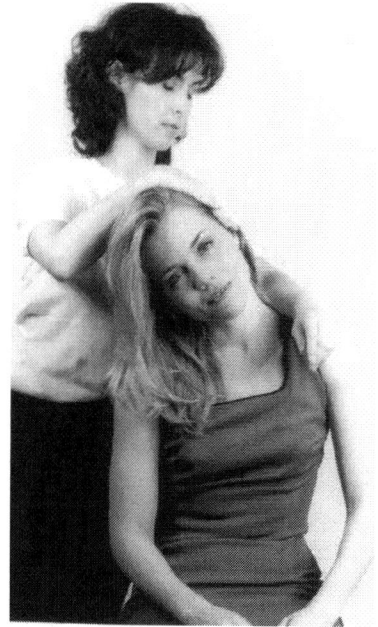

Levator Scapula Stretch

- Since most people have never heard of this muscles, trace your finger along their levator scapula so they have a sense of where they should feel the stretch

- Take the same starting position you used for the Trap Stretch, stabilizing the shoulder with your forearm. Start by asking them to drop their ear to their shoulder

- Then ask them to drop their head forward a little and turn their head to look toward their hip

- If they do not feel a stretch somewhere along the length of the levator scapula, place your hand on the back of the head and gently push their head toward their opposite hip, being sure to keep their shoulder stabilized

- Hold five to ten seconds and assist them in bringing their head upright

Variation

- If the person does not feel a stretch, here's a variation. Instead of stabilizing their shoulder with your forearm, lift their arm and place their hand on their shoulder blade as illustrated. This rotates the scapula and provides additional stretch.

- Make sure the upper arm is straight up and down. Then simply push the elbow gently downward toward the floor. While stabilizing the shoulder in this position, perform the stretch as outlined above

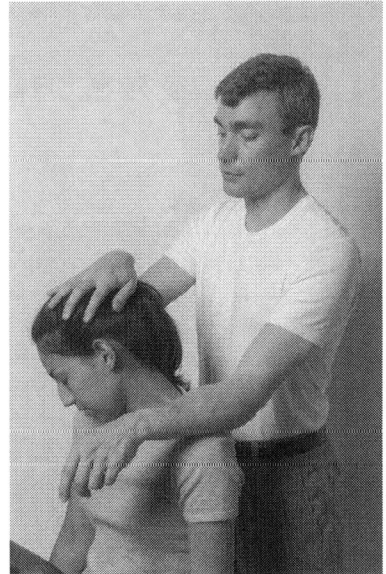

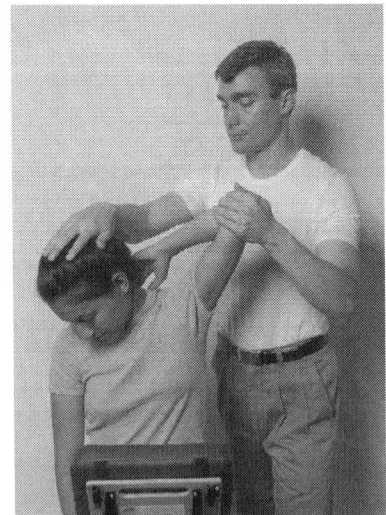

212

Bilateral Pec Stretch

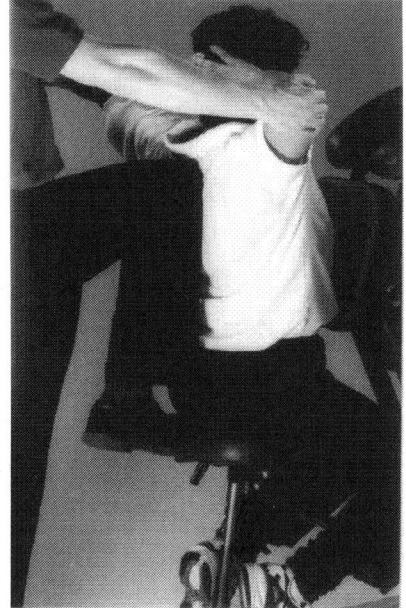

- Stand directly behind your partner

- Ask your partner to clasp both hands behind their head

- Ask your partner to slide forward slightly so that you may rest one foot on the edge of the chair

- With this knee, contact over the spine

- With both hands, contact each elbow and gently pull back straight towards you (your contact knee provides the support which prevents you from pulling the rest of their body backwards)

- If your knee and or your partner's spine is particularly bony, this may be uncomfortable

- This technique may increase the arch in some people's backs; as well, some people would not appreciate your foot on the chair

Unilateral Pec Stretch

- Stand directly behind your partner

- Ask you partner to place one hand behind their head; the elbow should be held high

- Put one hand directly on your partner's shoulder blade while the other holds their elbow

- As you pull your partner's elbow back, the hand stabilizing the shoulder blade applies a slight forward pressure; keep your arms relatively straight and let the movement come from your torso

- Ask your partner to communicate when they feel a stretch

- Hold for 5 seconds, encouraging them to breath slowly and deeply

- This is a good variation for a short practitioner coupled with a tall partner

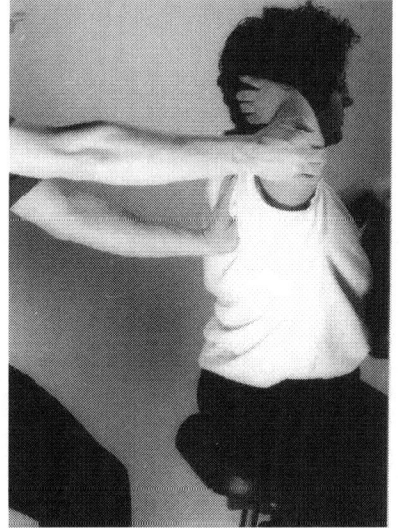

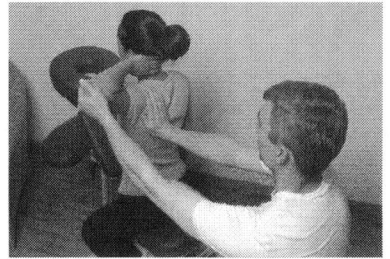

Backward Pec Stretch

- Stand directly behind your partner

- Ask your partner to clasp both hands behind their head

- Still standing behind your partner, turn yourself around so that your back is against their back

- Bring your arms over theirs so that their forearms are resting just beneath your armpit while your arms hang over (in this position you yourself would feel a stretch in your pectoralis muscles)

- From this position slowly and gently pull your arms forward which allows you to draw your partner's arms backward asking them to communicate when they feel a stretch

- Since you are not facing your partner during this stretch and cannot see their reaction, be sure to inform them that they should let you know immediately if anything feels uncomfortable

- This variation can be used for a tall practitioner working on a short customer.

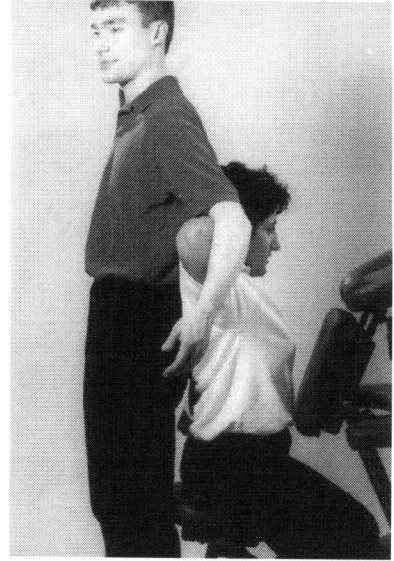

Customizing Your Massage

By combining various routine and accessory techniques you'll be able to customize your massage to meet both your needs and your client's preferences, whether that's a two-minute promotional massage or a one-hour, full-body chair massage. In this chapter you'll be provided with advice for accurately eliciting your client's preferences and be given guidelines for tailoring a massage to meet your client's needs in the best way possible.

So far, you've become proficient at a very structured 15-minute massage and you've learned a whole variety of additional techniques that cover the head, the toes and everything in between. You've even learned a few basic stretches that can be done in the chair.

Now it's time to put all these techniques together in your own massage sequences that are designed to meet the specific needs of each client. You'll be able to do a short two-minute massage on the ninth hole of a golf course or as a promotional test drive for your services. You'll also be able to do a full one hour massage with your client sitting in the chair. You'll find guidelines for doing this below.

If you have been learning the 15-minute routine from this book, the DVDs or in one of our live training programs, it's important to note that you'll need to shift gears. Don't get stuck in the timing, style or approach that you have been using to this point. You have lots of freedom to use everything you've learned in very different ways.

As mentioned previously, the 15-minute routine was designed for the corporate environment. The particular approach taken in putting this together may not be applicable to other situations or environments.

For example, the routine is 15-minutes long because from a sales perspective, to say that the service "takes no longer than a coffee break" is something corporate decision makers can relate to. However, if you are doing chair massage in someone's home, there is no reason why you can't do a full hour with the person sitting right in the chair.

As well, it was important that employees not get too relaxed. It was important to reduce their stress, but at the same time remain alert. So the routine is very fast-paced. You move from one technique to the other and there is very little repetition of any one technique. This constantly changing sensation creates a certain level of psycho-physiological arousal, as the brain has to continually orient to each new sensation. The person relaxes, but not as fully as if we were to massage more slowly and perform more sets and repetitions of each technique. If the massage were done in that way, the client's sensory system would have a chance to habituate to the sensation so their minds could really shut down.

There is no reason to be dogmatic about any particular approach. Your primary consideration should be ensuring that your client has a great experience and feels that their needs are met. So play around. Have some fun. As long as you stick to the simple guidelines below, it's hard to do it wrong.

Guidelines for customizing a relaxation massage

As with any massage, before you start it's important to do a thorough screening to determine that it is safe for your client to receive massage. As well, you'll want to identify any local contraindications so you can take that into consideration when designing your massage.

Make a Plan.

Before you start, decide what areas you are going to work on, what type of approach you are going to take, and what time frame you are going to work within. Base this plan on feedback from your client, including their current needs and preferences. It takes just a few minutes to find out about your clients preferences, but asking a few questions will allow you to perform a massage that will delight your client and make them feel taken care of.

There are some ways to ask questions that are more useful than others. The quality of your questions will determine the quality of their responses. If you ask something like, "Where would you like me to massage?" and they say, "My neck." what do you do? Do you just massage their neck? Are they going to be disappointed if you spend a little time massaging their hands? How much of a focus should you put on their neck?

Likewise, "What would you like me to do today?" isn't a good question for someone who is new to massage or who doesn't know your style of work. They see you as an expert and they are expecting you to have a thoughtful approach to their massage. Asking questions like that where you give responsibility for the treatment entirely to the client undermines your credibility as a professional.

One of the first pieces of information you'll want to determine is whether they've had any massage experiences in the past. You can simply ask: "Have you had massage before?

If they haven't, then you are working with a blank slate. You'll need to start off by finding out what their concerns and expectations are. You can ask questions like: "How's your body feeling today? Where do you typically hold your tension? Are there any areas in particular that you feel need attention?"

The answers to these questions should give you a general frame of reference. When customizing your massage for newbies, I'd suggest you do a variety of techniques throughout the upper body and arms. This gives the client a sense of how massage feels when performed on various regions. They'll also be better able to determine their preferences for their next massage as they now have an understanding for what's possible in terms of the range of techniques you can do.

If they have had massage in the past, they have a point of reference and can give you better information to help you come up with a plan that suits them. Two of the best questions to ask are, "What did you like?" and "What didn't you like?"

These open ended questions give you some valuable information to work with. Their answers will indicate their preferences in regards to the mechanics of the massage, like what areas they like having worked on and the level of pressure they prefer. As well, their answers also give us useful information about their overall experience of the massage.

For example, when you ask those questions you may get a response like, "I had a massage a few months ago. It felt so good on my neck. It hurt just little bit, but it was a good hurt. Do you know what I mean? I couldn't really relax though. The woman talked through the whole massage and I just wanted to enjoy the quiet."

In this case, you can determine that they enjoy work to their neck and like moderate to deep pressure. But you also know that they enjoy a quiet experience and that you should keep our interaction with them to a minimum while performing our massage.

If they give a vague answer like, "It was all good," then you may need to dig a little deeper. You can ask more probing questions like, "Is there anything that you really liked in particular? Are there any areas they massaged that felt particularly good? Was there anything they did that felt uncomfortable, unpleasant or that you would leave out of the massage if you could do it again?"

These are not closed questions, but they focus the response by helping the client think through their experience a little more carefully and force them to think about particular elements of their previous massages.

You can also ask, "Are there any particular areas that you'd like me to focus on today?" This gives them a chance to outline the areas they enjoy having massaged without precluding massage to other segments.

Lastly, you'll need to discuss the duration of the massage. This may have already been predetermined, ex. employees are booked into 15 minute time slots. If it hasn't, find out if they have any time restrictions. Many people choose chair massage because the sessions are short and can be scheduled between other tasks or appointments they may have. So if someone only has 20 minutes for their break, you want to make sure you can get through their session in that timeframe. Many therapists are generous and like to give their clients extra time in the chair. It's important that you keep your session within the timeframe you agreed on. If not, you may make them late for whatever is next on their agenda. This is bound to make them anxious and undo the benefits of your treatment. If you want to spend extra time with your client, be sure to ask them permission to do this to ensure this works for them.

If someone does not have limitations on the time they have available you can make suggestions based on what you feel is most appropriate for their circumstances and come to some agreement.

Based on all the information they've given you, you should have a general sense for their expectations and the type of approach you'll need to take when doing their massage.

Decide what areas you are going to massage and develop a rough time frame for each area based on their requirements and the agreed upon timeframe. It's good practice to review your plan with them in a general way before you start. Do this as part of the consent process. You can say something like:

"We have 20 minutes to do your massage and based on what you've told me, I'll think I'll start off with some general work to your back to get you relaxed. I'll focus a good portion of this massage on your neck and shoulders, which seem to be a little stiff from all the computer work you've been doing lately. Then I'm going to finish up with a few minutes on your hands. It's very relaxing. I'll use firm pressure throughout, but if it ever feels painful or uncomfortable please let me know right away. I can adjust my pressure for you. Does that sound good to you? Is there anything you'd like to do differently?"

Uncertainty, ambiguity and lack of control are highly co-related with stress and by removing these factors you set the stage for a relaxing and enjoyable experience. Having stated what you plan to do in this kind of way gives the client a good idea of what to expect for their massage. Knowing the sequence or approach in advance like this reduces any uncertainty they have about the process. For example, as you work on their back at the beginning of their session, they won't worry about whether or not you are going to massage their neck, which may be a concern for them.

Outlining your approach as part of the consent process also gives them a certain level of control. If they don't like certain elements of what you're suggesting or if they feel you don't understand what their needs are they have the opportunity to let you know.

Work In Segments

Think of your client's body in segments: neck, shoulders, arms, hands, mid-back, and low back, etc. You can further subdivide these segments, for example you can think of the back in quadrants, with right and left, upper and lower regions.

Thinking in segments like this will help you organize your massage sequence and ensure your timing is always spot on. From your initial discussion with your client, decide what areas are priorities for the client and be sure to focus on these segments.

Time Your Moves

One of the reasons for thinking in segments is that it allows you to manage your timing better. Develop a time frame for each area or segment. For example, with a five-minute massage, you may decide to spend 3 ½ minutes on the neck and shoulder segments and 1-½ minutes on the mid and lower back segments. You'll need to factor in some time for general introductory techniques, some superficial or broader techniques, which will allow the client some transition time as they begin to shift gears and get into a relaxation mode.

Have a clock or a watch at hand and stick to those time frames. By allotting specific time frames for each region you can ensure that you are consistent with the plan you received consent to implement for the client and you spend adequate time on the areas they wanted you to focus on.

Without being conscious about your timing in this way, it's easy to get caught up in working in certain areas that you like massaging or with particular techniques you personally prefer and fail to meet your client's needs. This is particularly true because the short time frames you're working within give you little room for errors like this.

Creating time frames for each segment is also important as you are beginning the process of learning how to customize your massage. The techniques are still fresh and not committed to memory yet, so the tendency is often to do the techniques you remember and move onto the next segment. Timing the amount of time you spend in any area and sticking to that time frame forces you better to memorize and apply the techniques you learned.

Complete One Segment before Moving onto the Next

Make sure you stick to the time you have allotted for an area and don't leave that segment until your time is up. This allows you to warm up the tissues and provides a sense of thoroughness or completeness for the client when working that area. The client habituates or gets used to the sensation in that area, which allows them to relax fully.

Moving back and forth from one area to another with each technique makes your massage feel erratic and rough. From the client perspective it doesn't feel like you know what you're doing. The person has no idea as to where they are going to be touched next and this puts them on edge. They are constantly surprised and can't fully relax.

If you draw a blank and feel that you can't remember enough techniques for the region you are working on, then simply slow down a little, do more sets of each technique and if necessary repeat techniques you've already done. The client doesn't know you've forgotten what you've learned in class and they won't care. In fact, the repetition makes the massage more relaxing.

When you don't massage a particular area for the time you've determined, you're deviating from the plan you outlined for your client. There's now a gap between what they expected and what's delivered. They'll be disappointed that you haven't given them the massage you promised.

Plan Your Transitions

As you learn how to do chair massage you are very focused on learning how to do the techniques themselves. You're focused on your positioning, your body use, getting your contact points right, palpating and targeting the right structures, etc.

Now, as you become more proficient with the techniques and start putting them together in various ways, it becomes equally or even more important to turn your focus towards the way you string the techniques together. In other words, your focus moves from the techniques to the spaces between the techniques.

Well executed transitions from one technique to the next and from one area of the body to another are what's going to set your massage apart from the others. So you can't let this happen by accident. You have to be very consciously aware of the way you make these transitions.

The notes I handle no better than many pianists. But the pauses between the notes – ah, that is where the art resides.
— *Artur Schnabel, one of the 20th century's great pianists*

As you developed a customized plan for your client's massage, think of the various segments of your client's body that you are going to massage and what order you're going to approach those. Organize the flow of the massage in your mind. For example, you may determine that you will do a couple of minutes of broad technique along the entire length of the back to start, do some massage to the shoulders bilaterally and then focus more specifically on the right shoulder and then the left shoulder before moving onto the neck. That's a fluid and logical sequence

Compare that to doing a massage where you start on one hand, do the other hand, move to the lower back, do several techniques to the neck and finish off with the arms. This doesn't seem to make sense in terms of a logical progression through the body. It seems like you're jumping haphazardly from one area to another. From a customer perspective it will feel odd and disjointed.

Before you begin your massage really think through the transitions you are going to make. Map it out so that there is no doubt in your mind as to where you are going next. Knowing in advance will allow you to maintain a fluid rhythm without interruption.

Besides thinking about which area you are going to transition to, it's important to consider exactly how you are going to make each transition. Sometimes it makes sense to give the customer a tactile cue. For example if you are transitioning from the back to the arm, slide one hand across the back and along the length of the arm as you gently grasp the wrist and elbow to lift the arm off the support and hang it down to their side. That kind of touch communicates exactly what you are going to do in a non-verbal way. There's no need to say that you're moving their arm. The signal is strong and the client understands instinctively what's happening and relaxes through the movement.

Don't feel that you have to do some kind of stroking motion to transition however. Sometimes the best way to move from one area to another is to be very direct. What becomes important in this case is not the tactile cue, but an even uninterrupted rhythm.

Besides thinking about the transition from one area to another you also need to consider the transitions from one technique to another. In most cases, the most important element in determining the fluidity of the transition will be your ability to maintain a constant rhythm as the change occurs.

The consistency in approach also plays a big role. Let's take for example, a transition from a compression technique to a percussion technique on the back. There is a significant potential to produce a jarring sensation with this kind of transition. In this case, as you start the percussion, be sure that the time between the compressions corresponds to the amount of time it takes to start the application of the percussion. Position your body beforehand so that you don't have to pause to adjust your stance and leave an unnecessarily long space which interrupts the flow or rhythm of the massage.

As well, the approach to the percussions has to simulate the approach of the compression as much as possible. You don't start by beating on them with all you've got. You try to maintain the sensation of a contact point that is similar to what you used for the compression. Likewise, the depth of the percussion should match what you used for the compression. Perform the percussions at exactly that depth and in the same place to give the client a moment to understand and settle into the transition and then you can start to gradually increase the depth or speed. This consistency in rhythm surface area, and depth allows the transition appear to be smooth and seamless even though the techniques are radically different in the way they are applied.

One common mistake in transitioning might best be described as "fluffing". Often practitioners will do a technique and then do a second or two of light stroking as a transition to the next technique. They do this repeatedly after each technique in an attempt to smooth the transition. In fact, they are doing the opposite. The radical change in sensation between, let's say, a deep compression technique and this light stroking is so extreme that the client can't help but become very aware of what's going on. From the perspective of the client it feels as though the practitioner has lost their rhythm and is trying to figure out what they are going to do next. It's like a tactile stutter.

Good transitions are not always about connecting techniques in a tactile way, but rather maintaining consistency in approach and rhythm.

Transitions are a lot like music in a movie. When well done, you aren't aware of the soundtrack that underlies the story. It enhances the emotion that exists without overpowering it. Likewise, your transitions from technique to technique and area to area should be invisible and simply enhance your client's experience of relaxation. They will only notice transitions when they are poorly done.

Think Two Techniques Ahead

As you become proficient in the techniques, you'll have to think less and less about their execution. You should always be aware of what your body is doing and how that is impacting the client, but the various elements become more automatic as the movement becomes ingrained in your nervous system. So as soon as you start performing one technique and start settling into the rhythm, shift your attention to the next technique you are going to do. This prevents you from hesitating as you finish that technique and allows you to transition smoothly into the next.

As you become increasingly comfortable with this and the technique you've learned in this textbook become part of your natural movement vocabulary, try to think ahead, not just to the next technique, but also to the technique that you plan to do after that. In other words, think at least two techniques ahead of where you are. This will make a big difference in the fluidity of your massage.

Use a Systematic Approach

If a client is unsure what is going to happen during their massage and what you're going to be doing to them, they will feel anxious on some level. A person will only relax to the extent that they know with certainty what to expect. To be deeply relaxing a massage must be predictable and unambiguous. Setting expectations happens before the massage in your verbal communication. However, in terms of informing your client what will happen next, even more communication happens in a non-verbal way through touch.

To make this tactile communication effective, you must develop a system for the application of the techniques that you can use consistently. If your approach is too haphazard, the client will not be able to sense what's coming next and will never fully relax.

However, when you use a consistent approach, the client is able to predict the general flow of the massage, even though it happens on a subconscious level.

In developing the standardized 15-minute routine outlined in this textbook, I used a very specific methodology when doing the routine. Approaches that I've incorporated in this routine include applying the techniques:

- Superior to inferior (sequencing movement from downwards)

- Proximal to distal (from the core outward)

- Right, then left

- Medial to lateral

- Superficial to deep

- Broad to specific (in terms of your contact point)

Watch the routine on video several times and you'll see with only a couple of exceptions, that this general approach is used through the entire sequence.

For example, when doing the Butterfly technique, you don't do the compressions downward along the spine and then back up the spine. Instead, when you reach the top of the pelvis you lift your hands and return them to the top of the back to begin another sequence that moves in a downward direction. Thus a pattern is developed.

Patterns are by their nature predictable. So your client has a very good sense, albeit unconsciously, where your hands are going to land next time they break contact with their body and they know the approach that you're going to take into their tissues. Nothing is a surprise. They can relax knowing exactly what to expect as you continue through various areas of their body.

Aim for Balance

Do the same massage to both sides of the body. Again, it helps the client to understand subconsciously what to expect and they will be better able to relax. By massaging both sides of the body equally and in exactly the same way the massage feels whole or complete.

There are three ways to approach this:

1. Work bilaterally (both sides at once)

This is built right into some techniques. For example, as you do the Butterfly technique down the back, one hand is place on each side of the spine.

2. Do one technique to one side and immediately repeat the technique to the other side

An example of this in the routine is doing a sequence of elbow compressions to the mid-back on one side and then immediately repeating the sequence on the other side.

3. Do a sequence of techniques to one side and repeat the exact sequence to the other side

This approach is illustrated in the arm sequence of the routine. In this case you can't physically massage both arms at the same time. Doing squeezes to a muscle on one side then running around the chair to do the same muscle on the other side doesn't make sense. It's too disruptive to the flow of the massage. So we do a series of techniques to the entire arm and hand, then repeat that exact same sequence to the opposite side.

Sometimes it can be very difficult to know where to begin when structuring a sequence of you own. To facilitate the process of going from a routine to completely customizing a massage it may be helpful to think of the routine as a framework and to simply build off of it. Here are a couple of exercises to help you do that:

1. Perform the routine, but after each routine technique is performed immediately do an accessory technique that targets the same area in the same way. So for example, after doing the *Gentle Circles*, do the *Sanding* technique. After doing the *Butterfly* do *Fist Walking*. To help you make these associations, take a sheet of paper and create two columns. Place the names of the routine techniques in the first column and in the second column list at least one accessory technique that corresponds to each routine technique.

2. Once you start to associate techniques in this way, then simply start replacing routine techniques for accessory techniques. You don't have to replace every one. Even if you replace just every second or third technique, you'll begin to intrinsically understand the range of options you have.

By using the routine as a framework like this you don't have to worry about the sequencing of your techniques, i.e. what areas are being massaged and in what order. Instead, you can focus on the techniques themselves and begin associating each technique with an area of the body.

Once you become more comfortable with using techniques this way, then you can start challenging yourself further by mixing up the sequence. For example, as an exercise you can try doing the routine backwards. It will still be familiar, but will help you shift your thinking about your approach and prevent you from using the routine sequence as a default.